# Study Guide

TO ACCOMPANY

1ST AUSTRALASIAN EDITION OF

# Nursing Research

## *Methods, Critical Appraisal and Utilisation*

**Doug Elliott and Gayle Burr**

**Kathleen Rose-Grippa and Mary Jo Gorney-Moreno**

Harcourt Mosby

Sydney Edinburgh London New York Philadelphia St Louis Toronto

[redacted]

Mosby
is a Harcourt Health Sciences Company

Harcourt Australia
30–52 Smidmore Street, Marrickville, NSW 2204

Harcourt Publishers International
24–28 Oval Road, London NW1 7DX

Harcourt Health Sciences
1–3 Baxter's Place, Leith Walk, Edinburgh EH1 3AF

Harcourt Health Sciences, The Curtis Centre
Independence Square West
Philadelphia PA 19106–3399

Harcourt Health Sciences
11830 Westline Industrial Drive
St Louis MO 63146



ISBN 1 875897 69 0

Publishing Editor: Vaughn Curtis
Publishing Services Manager: Helena Klijn
Edited by Brigid James, Writers Reign
Design Sarn Potter
Page make-up SPG
Printed in Australia by Mcpherson's Printing Group

# Contents


| | | |
|---|---|---|
| Acknowledgements | | iv |
| About the authors | | iv |
| Authors' note | | v |
| **Chapter 1** | From Research to Practice | 1 |
| **Chapter 2** | Overview of the Research Process | 4 |
| **Chapter 3** | Research Problems and Hypotheses | 6 |
| **Chapter 4** | Literature Review | 12 |
| **Chapter 5** | Theoretical Framework | 17 |
| **Chapter 6** | Legal and Ethical Issues | 22 |
| **Chapter 7** | Introduction to Design | 26 |
| **Chapter 8** | Quantitative Research Design | 30 |
| **Chapter 9** | Qualitative Approaches to Research: Methods and Sampling | 39 |
| **Chapter 10** | Sampling | 45 |
| **Chapter 11** | Data Collection Methods | 49 |
| **Chapter 12** | Reliability and Validity in Quantitative Research | 57 |
| **Chapter 13** | Qualitative Approaches to Research: Data Collection, Analysis and Interpretation | 62 |
| **Chapter 14** | Descriptive Data Analysis | 65 |
| **Chapter 15** | Inferential Data Analysis | 71 |
| **Chapter 16** | Analysis of the Findings | 74 |
| **Chapter 17** | Evaluating the Qualitative Research Report | 79 |
| **Chapter 18** | Evaluating Quantitative Research Studies | 83 |
| **Chapter 19** | Research Utilisation | 85 |
| References | | 90 |
| Appendix | | 93 |

# Acknowledgements

The authors acknowledge Ms Maria Apostol for typing early drafts of the manuscript. Acknowledgement is also made to Vaughn Curtis and Brigid James for publishing and editorial direction and support.

# About the authors

Doug Elliott is Associate Professor and Head of Department, Department of Clinical Nursing at the University of Sydney. Dr Gayle Burr is a senior lecturer in the Department of Clinical Nursing, also at the University of Sydney.

# Authors' note

This Study Guide was designed to accompany the textbook *Nursing Research: Methods, Critical Appraisal and Utilisation* by Geri Lo-Biondo-Wood and Judith Haber; Australasian edition by Christine Beanland and Zevia Schneider. As with the textbook, this learning resource was adapted in part from the Study Guide created by Kathleen Rose-Grippa and Mary Jo Gorney-Moreno which accompanies the United States' version of the textbook.

The Guide mirrors the chapter framework of *Nursing Research*, includes activities directed to the articles reprinted in the appendices and the body of the text, and uses examples from Australian and New Zealand studies as well as the wider international literature. Students are encouraged to improve their knowledge and skills in research utilisation through reading the text and completion of the associated activities. Each chapter in the Study Guide provides learning objectives, activities with answers in the appendix, and related activities or a post-test.

# 1 From Research to Practice

It is important that students have an understanding of the role of research in nursing. The *Nursing Research* textbook provides a background, both historical and contextual, for students to consider while completing the following activities.

## Learning outcomes

On completion of this chapter the student should be able to do the following:

- understand beginning research terminology
- identify the links between nursing research, theory, education and practice
- consider the current and future role of research in the nursing discipline.

## ACTIVITY ONE

Match the phrase in Column A with the appropriate term in Column B. Each term is used only once. It may be useful to review the glossary in the textbook.

**COLUMN A**

- Systematic inquiry into possible relationships among particular phenomena
- One who reads critically and applies research findings in nursing practice
- Examines the effects of nursing care on patient outcomes in a systematic process
- A critical evaluation of a research report's content and scientific merit based on a set of criteria
- Implementation of a scientifically sound research-based innovation into clinical practice
- Theoretical or pure research that generates, tests and expands theories that explain phenomena

**COLUMN B**

**a** critique
**b** consumer
**c** research
**d** clinical evaluation
**e** basic research
**f** research utilisation



## ACTIVITY TWO

This activity is designed for students to consider, individually, in pairs or in groups, the issue of nursing research within the broader context of nursing practice and the nursing discipline.

**a** List and discuss the various roles of nurses.

**b** What is your honest opinion about the purpose and value of nursing research?

**c** Conduct a SWOB analysis of nursing research. Brainstorm the issues and categorise them accordingly:

| Strengths | Opportunities |
|---|---|
| | |
| **Weaknesses** | **Barriers** |
| | |

**d** What are the benefits or potential benefits of nursing research for clinical practice?

**e** How can nursing research be translated into practice?

## ACTIVITY THREE

The Royal College of Nursing, Australia (RCNA) developed a position statement on Nursing Research in 1998 (see page 5 of the textbook). Obtain a copy of the statement through your campus library, the RCNA (http://www.rcna.org.au/) or speak to your tutor.

**a** As a student of nursing, what is your response to the RCNA's belief about nursing research?

**b** Do you agree with the recommendations from the RCNA?

**c** Are these recommendations achievable?

## ACTIVITY FOUR

The textbook identifies three scholarly journals which are predominantly sourced from Australia.

**a** Access a copy of each of the following journals and find out their aims and scope: *Contemporary Nurse; International Journal of Nursing Practice; Nursing Inquiry.*

**b** What other Australasian-based nursing journals are published?

There is no post-test for this chapter. Consider the critical thinking challenges on page 18 of the textbook.

# 2 Overview of the Research Process

The following activities are designed to introduce the process of critical reading when reviewing research articles.

## Learning outcomes

On completion of this chapter the student should be able to do the following:

- consider the components and process of critical reading
- use beginning strategies for the critical reading of research articles
- differentiate between the format and style of qualitative and quantitative research articles.

## ACTIVITY ONE

Determine whether the article in Appendix D in the textbook (Dracup et al., 1997) is a quantitative or qualitative study.

You can utilise the following points to determine if the study is of a quantitative design. First answer yes or no for each item, then summarise your thoughts in a paragraph.

**a** Hypotheses are stated or implied in the article. Yes No

**b** The terms 'control' and 'treatment group' appear. Yes No

**c** The terms 'survey', 'correlational', or 'ex post facto' are used. Yes No
(Note: Read the glossary definitions for help in answering this question.)

**d** The terms 'random' or 'convenience' are mentioned in relation to the sample. Yes No

**e** Variables are measured by instruments or tools. Yes No

**f** Reliability and validity of instruments are discussed. Yes No

**g** Statistical analyses are used. Yes No

**h** Write a summary.

## ACTIVITY TWO

You are reading the Kermode (1995) article in Appendix C in the textbook and find a citation to 'Colaizzi's method' of theme identification. You have never heard about this data analysis method before, but believe that you could understand the article better if you could learn about it. How will you quickly find out about this method?

## ACTIVITY THREE

To read a research study critically, the reader must have skilled reading, writing and reasoning abilities. Read the abstract for the study by Webb and Koch (1997), partly presented on page 37 of the textbook using the following questions.

**a** What concepts can you identify?

**b** Are there any unfamiliar concepts or terms that you would need to clarify? List them.

**c** Were the assumptions or rationale for the study appropriate?

## POST-TEST

Read the extracts from the study by Wellard and Palaster (1996) presented on pages 37–9 of the textbook.

**a** What concepts can you identify?

**b** Are there any unfamiliar concepts or terms that you would need to clarify? List them.

**c** What assumptions or rationale would you question?

# 3 Research Problems and Hypotheses

The problem statement and hypothesis are very important. If presented correctly, a problem statement can be very helpful to you as a consumer of nursing research because it concisely describes the essence of the study. The hypothesis or research question provides the most succinct link between the underlying theoretical base and the research design. Thus, its analysis is pivotal to the analysis of the entire study.

## Learning outcomes

On completion of this chapter the student should be able to do the following:

- define terms related to the problem statement and hypothesis
- differentiate between the characteristics of research problems and hypotheses
- distinguish between a research hypothesis, statistical hypothesis, research question, directional hypothesis, and non-directional hypothesis
- identify independent and dependent variables
- apply critiquing criteria to the evaluation of a problem statement in a research report.

## ACTIVITY ONE

A good problem statement exhibits four characteristics. Read the problem statements below (the first four are also listed on page 61 of the textbook) and examine them to determine if each of the four criteria is present. Following each problem statement is a list representing the four criteria. Circle yes or no to indicate whether each criterion is met.

The problem statement:

i clearly and unambiguously identifies the variables under consideration

ii clearly expresses the variables' relationship to each other

iii specifies the nature of the population being studied

iv implies the possibility of empirical testing.

**a** *The purpose of this study was to describe prehospital delay time in Australian patients experiencing symptoms of evolving acute MI and to identify the cognitive, emotional, socio-demographic, and clinical factors which contribute to this delay (Dracup et al., 1997).*

i Yes No
ii Yes No
iii Yes No
iv Yes No

**b** *The study aims to (1) supplement previous quantitative investigations into childhood immunisation uptake rates; (2) to explore the beliefs of primary child caregivers about common childhood diseases and related immunisations; and (3) offer some explanation as to the possible constraints affecting uptake of childhood immunisations (White & Thomson, 1995).*

i Yes No
ii Yes No
iii Yes No
iv Yes No

**c** *The aim of this study was to assess how nurses and doctors record alcohol histories on patients and the frequency and appropriateness of their use of an alcohol-withdrawal scale in an acute hospital setting (Burns & Adams, 1997).*

i Yes No
ii Yes No
iii Yes No
iv Yes No

**d** *This research attempts to develop a reliable and valid questionnaire to assess midwives' attitudes to the cognitive abilities of pregnant women and also, appropriate educational experiences for the women (Jackson et al., 1996).*

i Yes No
ii Yes No
iii Yes No
iv Yes No

**e** *The purpose of this study was to describe the association between the marital relationship and the health of the wife with chronic fatigue and immune dysfunction syndrome (CFIDS) (Goodwin, 1997).*

i Yes No
ii Yes No
iii Yes No
iv Yes No

**f** *This study examined the effects of an individualised computerised testing system for baccalaureate nursing students enrolled in health assessment and obstetrics-women's health during a 3-year period (Bloom & Trice, 1997).*

i Yes No
ii Yes No
iii Yes No
iv Yes No

**g** *This study was an examination of perceptions about the causes of coronary artery disease and the timeline of the disease among 105 patients hospitalised because of myocardial infarction or for coronary angiography and receiving the diagnosis of coronary artery disease (Zerwic, King & Wlasowicz, 1997).*

i Yes No
ii Yes No
iii Yes No
iv Yes No



## ACTIVITY TWO

The ability to distinguish between independent and dependent variables is a crucial preliminary step when determining whether or not a research hypothesis is a succinct statement of the relationship between two variables. Identify the variables in the following examples. Decide which is the independent (presumed cause or explanatory) variable and which is the dependent (presumed effect or outcome) variable.

**a** The use of cathode ray terminals (CRTs) increases the incidence of birth defects.

**b** Individuals with birth defects have a higher incidence of independence–dependence conflicts than individuals without birth defects.

**c** What is the relationship between daily moderate consumption of white wine and serum cholesterol levels?

**d** Problem-oriented recording leads to more effective patient care than narrative recording.

**e** Nurses and physicians differ in the way they view the extended-role concept for nurses.

**f** What is the extent to which sex, age, height and weight predict the following physiological outcomes: forced expiratory volume in one second (FEV1), haemoglobin concentration, food intake, serum glucose concentration, total serum cholesterol?

## ACTIVITY THREE

Take each hypothesis (or research question) from Activity Two and label it with the appropriate abbreviation from the key provided. More than one abbreviation from the key may be used to describe each item.

***Key***

| | |
|---|---|
| DH | Directional hypothesis |
| NDH | Non-directional hypothesis |
| Hr | Research hypothesis |
| RP | Research problem |
| RQ | Research question |
| Ho | Statistical hypothesis |

## ACTIVITY FOUR

The next step is to practise writing different types of hypotheses. Return to the first three of the six hypotheses/questions/problems which you labelled in Activity Three as a specific type of hypothesis, research question or problem statement. Rewrite each of the first three to meet the conditions of the remaining types of questions or hypotheses. The first one is partially completed to provide an example.

**a** The use of cathode ray terminals (CRTs) increases the incidence of birth defects.

| | |
|---|---|
| DH | The use of CRTs increases the incidence of birth defects. |
| NDH | The use of CRTs influences the incidence of birth defects. |
| Hr | The use of CRTs increases the incidence of birth defects. |
| RP | |
| RQ | |
| Ho | |

**b** Individuals with birth defects have a higher incidence to independence–dependence conflicts than individuals without birth defects.

DH
NDH
Hr
RP
RQ
Ho

**c** What is the relationship between daily moderate consumption of white wine and serum cholesterol levels?

DH
NDH
Hr

RP
RQ
Ho

## ACTIVITY FIVE

Critique the following hypotheses which were both tested in a study by Beck et al., 1997.

### *Hypothesis 1*

*There will be significant improvement in the dressing independence of cognitively impaired nursing-home residents following implementation of strategies to promote independence in dressing (SPID).*

| | | | |
|---|---|---|---|
| **a** | Is the hypothesis clearly stated in a declarative form? | Yes | No |
| **b** | Are the independent and dependent variables identified in the statement of the hypothesis? | Yes | No |
| **c** | Are the variables measurable or potentially measurable? | Yes | No |
| **d** | Is the hypothesis stated in such a way that it is testable? | Yes | No |
| **e** | Is the hypothesis stated objectively without value-laden words? | Yes | No |
| **f** | Is the direction of the relationship in the hypothesis clearly stated? | Yes | No |
| **g** | Is each of the hypotheses specific to one relationship so that each hypothesis can be either supported or not supported? | Yes | No |



### *Hypothesis 2*

*There will be no difference in the time required by nursing assistants to complete dressing activities with cognitively impaired nursing-home residents before and after implementing strategies to promote independence in dressing.*

| | | | |
|---|---|---|---|
| **a** | Is the hypothesis clearly stated in a declarative form? | Yes | No |
| **b** | Are the independent and dependent variables identified in the statement of the hypothesis? | Yes | No |
| **c** | Are the variables measurable or potentially measurable? | Yes | No |
| **d** | Is the hypothesis stated in such a way that it is testable? | Yes | No |
| **e** | Is the hypothesis stated objectively without value-laden words? | Yes | No |
| **f** | Is the direction of the relationship in the hypothesis clearly stated? | Yes | No |
| **g** | Is each of the hypotheses specific to one relationship so that each hypothesis can be either supported or not supported? | Yes | No |

## ACTIVITY SIX

How do you determine whether a sentence is a problem statement or a hypothesis?

## POST-TEST

Choose the terms from the key provided which best describe items **a–g**. More than one abbreviation from the key may be used to describe each item.

***Key***

| | |
|---|---|
| RH | Research question |
| DH | Directional hypothesis |
| NDH | Non-directional hypothesis |
| Hr | Research hypothesis |
| Ho | Statistical hypothesis |

**a** There will be no change in self-rated body image among women in the three patient groups.

**b** What is the relationship between organisational climate dimensions and job satisfaction of nurses in neonatal intensive care units?

**c** The higher the perceived parental support, the lower the girls' general fearfulness.

**d** There will be a significant difference in pre-post changes in cognitive development level between undergraduate nursing students who have completed a research course and those who have not.

**e** The post-test mean of selected psychological variables for the experimental group will be lower than that of the control group.

**f** There will be no association found between the level of social support and self-care health practices.

**g** What is the level of post-operative infection following the use of clean tracheostomy care?

# 4 Literature Review

The term 'review of the literature' most commonly refers to that section of a research study in which the researcher describes the link between previously existing knowledge and the current study. Other research-related uses of a review of the literature include:

- developing an overall impression of what research and clinical work has been done in a given area
- assisting in the clarification of the research problem
- polishing research design ideas
- finding possible data collection and data analysis strategies.

## Learning outcomes

On completion of this chapter, the student should be able to do the following:

- identify purposes of the literature review for research and non-research activities
- identify those paragraphs in any research study that constitute the literature review
- distinguish between primary and secondary sources
- differentiate between conceptual and data-based literature
- evaluate the degree to which relevant concepts and variables are discussed in the literature review
- compare the advantages and disadvantages of CD-ROM and Internet databases with print databases
- critically analyse the types of information available on the World Wide Web (WWW).

## ACTIVITY ONE

What is the relationship between a review of the literature and nursing research, education and practice?

## ACTIVITY TWO

Summarise the main points that reflect the purposes of a literature review from the research consumer's perspective.

## ACTIVITY THREE

Following is a list of terms and examples describing either conceptual or data-based literature. Decide whether each example describes conceptual literature (C) or data-based literature (D). Refer to Tables 4.5 and 4.7 of the textbook for help.

**a** Published qualitative studies.

**b** Published articles or books discussing theories or concepts.

**c** Unpublished abstracts of research studies from research conferences.

**d** Published studies in journals describing relationships between variables.

**e** *The purpose was to introduce the symptom interpretation model (SIM) and facilitate understanding symptoms from an intrapersonal perspective. Theory derivation was used to develop SIM for understanding comparisons of known and new symptoms in a behavioural outcomes context (Teel et al., 1997).*

**f** *The objective of this study was to evaluate the effect of placebo and 'active' muscle stimulation in the rehabilitation of quadriceps muscle function in patients with osteoarthritis of the knee. All subjects were recruited from a waiting list for knee joint replacement (Oldham & Howe, 1997).*

## ACTIVITY FOUR

Researchers who are also clinicians are generally interested in solving clinical problems regardless of whether the solution is for immediate or future use. When faced with a problem in clinical practice it is important to find out what others have learned about it. To do this it is necessary to firstly go to the nursing literature. List five nursing journals that publish reports or research studies that a clinician might use to find out more about a problem.

## ACTIVITY FIVE

The review of the literature is usually easy to find. Generally one of the early sections of the report (even if the report is abridged) is labelled 'Review of literature' or 'Relevant literature' or some other comparable term.

Note: The length of the literature review section in a journal varies. A range from two to several paragraphs is the most common.

**a** Examine the articles in Appendix A (Barclay et al., 1996) and Appendix D (Dracup et al., 1997) of the textbook. Comment briefly on the way in which the review of the literature is presented in each article.

**b** Does the literature review in each of the above articles uncover gaps or inconsistencies in knowledge? If yes, explain what gap or inconsistency is identified.

**c** Determine how recent the articles listed in the references section of the article by Dracup et al. (1997) are. Do they portray the development of the research over time?

**d** A good literature review should read like a story. For example, there may initially be qualitative studies that attempt to identify which variables are important to the problem or paradigm. At some point you should also see researchers progressively analyse each of the variables, gradually narrowing and defining the scope of the problem. Others might continue to look at the problem qualitatively. Can this approach be seen in the literature review and reference section of the Dracup et al. (1997) article?

**e** Critique the currency of the references. Write the story you see in the reference section and as described in the review of the literature.



## ACTIVITY SIX

Sometimes it is difficult to understand the distinction between primary and secondary sources of information. The following comparison may be helpful. If you are considering giving a patient an injection for pain, whose report would you feel most comfortable evaluating – the report of a family member or nurse's aide (that is, secondary source) or the actual report by the patient (that is, primary source)?

As a consumer of nursing research, it is important to evaluate the credibility of research designs and reports based in part on whether they are generated from primary or secondary sources so that you know whether the information you are reading is a first-hand report or someone else's interpretation of the material.

**a** The following words or phrases describe either primary or secondary sources. Indicate those describing primary (P) and those describing secondary (S) sources.

- summaries of research studies
- first-hand accounts
- biographies
- textbooks
- patient records
- reports written by the researcher
- dissertations or master's theses

**b** The best source for primary research studies is the WWW. True False

**c** The CINAHL Print Index must be used for literature searches of material before which year?

**d** Which is the best database for a search of nursing literature? Why?

- MEDLINE
- CINAHL

**e** Log onto the Internet through your campus library, computer laboratory or at home if you have access. Use a search engine, for example, Netscape Navigator or Internet Explorer (see page 102 of the textbook) to find:

- the URL (location address) for *The Australian Electronic Journal of Nursing Education*
- the location of the most recent review of best practice from the Joanna Briggs Institute of Evidence Based Nursing and Midwifery
- the title of the Home Page with the URL http://ublib.buffalo.edu/libraries/units/hsl/internet/nsgsites.html

**f** *The Online Journal of Knowledge Synthesis for Nursing* can provide access to current, synthesised research. Use the CINAHL database to identify the authors of the article entitled 'Factors related to adult patient decision making about withholding or withdrawing nutrition and/or hydration' published in 1999.

**g** You have noticed an increased incidence of bedsores on your ward and decide to search the literature for the latest information on prevention and treatment. Identify at least three key words/phrases that you could use to begin the search.



## ACTIVITY SEVEN

Below is a selected list of references from the Dracup et al., (1997) article in Appendix D in the textbook. Indicate whether the reference is conceptual (C) or data-based (D), and whether it is primary (P) or secondary (S).

**a** Leitch JW, Birbara T, Freedman B et al.: Factors influencing the time from onset of chest pain to arrival at the hospital, *Med J Aust* 150:6–8, 1989.

**b** Bandura A: Self-efficacy: toward a unifying theory of behavior change, *Psychol Bull* 84:191–198, 1977.

**c** Bailey WC, Richards JM Jr, Brooks CM et al.: A randomised trial to improve self-management practices of adults with asthma, *Arch Intern Med* 150:1664–67, 1990.

**d** Fibrinolytic Therapy Trialists' (FTT) Collaborative Group: Indications for fibrinolytic therapy in suspected acute myocardial infarction: collaborative overview of early mortality and major morbidity results from all randomized trials of more than 1000 patients, *Lancet* 343:311–22, 1994.

**e** Dracup K, Moser D, Eisenberg M et al.: Causes of delay in seeking treatment for symptoms of acute myocardial infarction, *Soc Sci Med* 40:379–92, 1995.

## ACTIVITY EIGHT

Many health care professionals and consumers now use the WWW to search for health care information. Before using the WWW, develop a set of questions that would be useful to critique the scientific merit of health care information obtained in this way. List at least five questions.

It may be helpful to recall what you have learned about the peer-review process before journal articles are accepted for publication, and to review the critiquing criteria in the textbook.

## POST-TEST

**1** Indicate whether the following are examples of primary (P) or secondary (S) sources.

**a** This article reviews the published literature on the effectiveness of cardiac rehabilitation in terms of improving mortality, quality of life, and employment in those with myocardial infarction and stable angina pectoris (Pell, 1997).

**b** The purpose was to describe the lived experience of post-operative pain in frail, elderly women using Colaizzi's (1978) phenomenological approach (Zalon, 1997).

**2** Turn to the reference section in the Barclay et al. (1996) article in Appendix A in the textbook, which is partially reproduced below. Indicate whether it is conceptual (C) or data-based (D), and whether it is primary (P) or secondary (S).

**a** Zayas LH: Psychodynamic and developmental aspects of expectant and new fatherhood: clinical derivatives from the literature, *Clinical Social Work Journal* 15(1): 8–21, 1987.

**b** Imle M: Third trimester concerns of expectant parents in transition to parenthood, *Holistic Nursing Practice* 4(3): 25–36, 1990.

**c** Barclay L, McDonald P, O'Loughlin JA: Sexuality and pregnancy – an interview study, *The Australian and New Zealand Journal of Obstetrics and Gynaecology* 34(1): 1–7, 1994.

**d** Nyamathi A, Shuler P: Focus group interview: a research technique for informed nursing practice, *Journal of Advanced Nursing* 15: 1281–88, 1990.

**3** Differentiate between 'refereed' and 'non-refereed' journals.

**4** What are the advantages of using computer databases as well as print databases when doing a literature search?

**5** Literature reviews are usually presented in a) chronological order or b) according to the variables being studied. Examine the four articles in the appendices of the textbook and comment on the presentation (a or b) of each literature review.

**6** Given that 'primary resources are essential for literature reviews', what is the value of secondary resources?

# 5 Theoretical Framework

It is not uncommon for the beginning research consumer to find the theoretical part of a study difficult. However, the theoretical framework of a study provides the reader with the opportunity to see the research problem in its context. The task when critiquing this section of a study is to consider the researcher's perspective and then ask the following questions:

- How clear is the researcher's argument?
- Does the theoretical framework connect all of the components of the study?
- Is there a clear relationship between the theoretical discussion and application to clinical practice?

## Learning outcomes

On completion of this chapter the student should be able to do the following:

- discuss the following terms in relation to their distinguishing characteristics: concept, construct, theoretical framework, conceptual definition, operational definition, variable
- define inductive and deductive thinking
- identify the major concepts in a given study
- evaluate the relationship of a given theoretical framework to the relevant study and to clinical practice.

## ACTIVITY ONE

Write down in your own words the defining characteristics of:

- inductive thinking
- deductive thinking.

## ACTIVITY TWO

As explained in the textbook, concepts are the building blocks of a study. The greater the ease with which you can identify concepts, the easier it will become to analyse the theoretical framework of a given study. Once you can perform this analysis, you will be able to follow the line of logic from problem to conclusions.

Identify the concepts in each of the following excerpts from research:

**a** *A theoretical model was developed and tested to explain the effects of learned helplessness, self-esteem, and depression on the health practices of homeless women (Flynn, 1997).*

**b** *... to examine the relationships among illness, uncertainty, stress, coping, and emotional well-being at the time of entry into a clinical drug trial (Wineman et al., 1996).*

**c** *As part of a larger study of the impact of a social support intervention on pregnancy outcome for lower-income African-American women ... (Bolla et al., 1996).*



**d** *... to identify determinants of violent and non-violent behavior among a group of vulnerable inner-city youths (Powell, 1997).*

**e** *... prevalence and consequences of verbal abuse of staff nurses by physicians were examined in the context of Lazarus' stress-coping model (Manderino & Berkey, 1997).*

## ACTIVITY THREE

Choose one concept from each of the five research examples presented in Activity two.

**a** In your own words write a definition of the chosen concept.

**b** Compare your definition of the chosen concept with the definition of the same concept written by one of your peers. How close were the two definitions? Think about the similarities and differences. Assume the two of you were going to work as co-investigators on a study to investigate the concept.

- What would you need to resolve?
- Look again at the concepts. Do any of them closely resemble a construct?

## ACTIVITY FOUR

Identify the conceptual and/or operational definitions for the studies presented in each of the four appendices in the textbook. Do not expect every study to include both. It is also possible that some definitions are implicit rather than explicit.

## ACTIVITY FIVE

The following activity provides an initial look at how theory, concepts, definitions, variables and hypotheses fit together. There is more detail about variables and hypotheses in a later chapter. The focus here is on understanding how they are based in theory.

Match the terms in Column B with the appropriate definition or example in Column A. Words in bold print in Column A indicate the element to be matched to a term. Items in Column B may be used more than once.

### COLUMN A

**a** ***Fatigue symptoms were measured using the Modified Fatigue Symptoms Checklist (MFSC), a list of 30 symptoms of fatigue. Scores range from zero (no fatigue symptoms) to 30 symptoms (maximum fatigue)*** (Milligan, Flenniken & Pugh, 1996)

**b** ***... stress and empowerment were used to guide this study*** (Kendra, 1996)

**c** *Serenity is viewed as a* ***learned, positive emotion of inner peace that can be sustained, that decreases perceived stress and improves physical and emotional health*** (Roberts & Whall, 1996)

**d** ***Older (that is more than 35 years old) first-time mothers*** (Reese & Harkless, 1996)

**e** ***Clinical decision-making***

**f** ***Quality of life***

**g** *Acute confusion is a transient syndrome characterized primarily by* ***abnormalities in attention and cognition, but disordered psychomotor behavior, sleep-wake disturbance, and autonomic nervous system disturbances*** *are not uncommon* (Neelon et al., 1996)

**h** *Are there* ***breathing pattern*** *changes from test to test or from the beginning to the end of the test?* (Hopp et al., 1996)

**i** ***The combination of injury experience, knowledge, demographic, health beliefs, and social influence variables will predict home hazard accessibility*** (Russell & Champion, 1996)

### COLUMN B

- variable
- hypothesis
- construct
- operational definition
- concept
- conceptual definition

## ACTIVITY SIX

This activity gives you the opportunity to use all of the thinking you have done so far in tracing a variable from the introduction of a study through the theoretical rationale of that same study. Read the first part of the Waldenström and Nilsson (1994) study in Appendix B of the textbook to the section entitled 'Methods'. Do not read the methods section.

**a** Name the major variables in this study. (Read the title closely for this information.)

**b** Read the next paragraphs and summarise three factors that you have learnt about breastfeeding and three factors about delivery care.

**c** What type of reasoning is operating in this study?

**d** Were hypotheses developed for this study?

**e** Would you describe the theoretical rationale for this study as:

- a theoretical framework
- a theory
- a conceptual model
- none of the above.

**f** What is the clinical concern that is the basis of this study?

## POST-TEST



1 List three reasons supporting the importance of the theoretical rationale of a study.

2 Read each statement. Decide if the statement is true (T) or false (F). Rewrite the false statements to make them true statements.

**a** 'Caregiving' is an example of a concept that is so clearly understood there is no need for it to be operationally defined in a research study.

**b** The following definition is an example of a conceptual definition:

*The Beck Dressing Performance Scale (BDPS) (Beck, 1988) was used to measure the major dependent variable, the level of caregiver assistance provided during dressing. The dressing function is broken down into 42 discrete component steps for males and 45 for females. A trained rater assigns each step of the dressing activity a score of 0 (independent) to 7 (complete dependence) based on the amount of assistance required to complete each step. Higher scores indicate greater dependence (Beck et al., 1997).*

**c** The words in bold in the following phrase are the name of a construct:

*... **define a professional practice model (PPM)** as a system that supports registered nurse control over the delivery of nursing care and the environment in which care is delivered (Hoffart & Woods, 1997).*

**d** The following is an example of a conceptual definition:

*Although there is no standard definition of social support, there seems to be general acceptance of some basic typologies. House, Umberson and Landis (1988) defined social support as positive dimensions of relationships that may promote health and buffer stress (Bolla et al., 1996).*

**e** The following is a sketch of a concept:

*... verbal abuse was defined as verbal behaviors that are perceived as humiliating, degrading, and/or disrespectful. Because verbally abusive encounters potentially can be stressful, it seemed appropriate to address this issue within the framework of a model of stress ... the major tenet of this model [sic: Lazarus' transactional model of stress coping] is that stress occurs in the face of perceived demands that tax or exceed the perceived coping resources of the person (Manderino & Berkey, 1997).*

# 6 Legal and Ethical Issues

Patient advocacy is one of the primary roles of a professional nurse. Nowhere is this more necessary than in the field of research. The nurse must be the client advocate, whether acting as the researcher, a participant in data gathering or a provider of care for research subjects. A multitude of legal and ethical issues exist in research. Nurses must be aware of, assess and evaluate these issues. They also need to be knowledgeable about the purpose and functions of Institutional Ethics Committees and the government regulations on which they are based.

## Learning outcomes

On completion of this chapter the student should be able to do the following:

- identify the essential elements of an informed consent form
- describe the Institutional Ethics Committee's role in the research review process
- describe the nurse's role as a patient advocate in research situations
- critique the ethical aspects of a research study.

## ACTIVITY ONE

**a** Explain why the principle 'the ends justify the means' cannot be tolerated in the conduct of research that involves human subjects.

**b** What organisation is responsible for the guidelines for the ethical conduct of research involving human subjects in Australia?

**c** What were the guidelines based upon?

**d** How can the guidelines be accessed?

**e** What is the role and function of Institutional Ethics Committees?

**f** What are the main areas of research that create discussion, controversy and debate at present and will continue in the future?

**g** What are the rights of human subjects involved in a research project?

## ACTIVITY TWO

List the three ethical principles relevant to the conduct of research involving human subjects.

## ACTIVITY THREE

Review the articles in Appendices A–D of the textbook. For each article, describe if and how informed was obtained and how the author described obtaining permission from the Institutional Ethics Committee or other relevant organisation.



## ACTIVITY FOUR

Identify at least four groups of subjects who are vulnerable or have diminished autonomy.

## ACTIVITY FIVE

Read the following study excerpts as if you are a nurse member of an Institutional Ethics Committee. List any conditions that might require special circumstances.

**a** *The study examined the effect of an individualised computerised testing system for [undergraduate] nursing students enrolled in health assessment and obstetrics/women's health during a 3-year period. One hundred and twenty-seven students participated in the study. The testing software, Pedagogue ™, was used to generate the computer test, and the students took all quizzes on-line. The mean score on computer tests in both courses were as good as, or better than previous scores on paper-pencil forms of the tests (p<.05) (Bloom & Trice, 1997).*

**b** *Inner-city male adolescents in jail in New York City (N = 427) were interviewed to examine correlates of cocaine or crack use. Twenty-three percent has used cocaine or crack in the month before arrest and 32% reported lifetime use. Substantial rates of robbery, murder, other violent crime, weapons possession, and drug dealing were found. However, type of crime, including violent crime, was not related either to cocaine/crack use or to drug dealing. Current cocaine/crack users were more likely to use alcohol, marijuana, and intranasal heroin; to have multiple previous arrests; to be out of school; to be psychologically distressed; to have been* *sexually molested as a child; to have substance-abusing parents; and to have cocaine/crack-using friends. They were also more likely to have frequent sex with girls, to be gay or bisexual, and to engage in anal intercourse. The findings should be considered in developing more effective drug abuse prevention and treatment interventions, and HIV prevention and education for incarcerated at-risk adolescents (Kang, Magura & Shapiro, 1994).*

## ACTIVITY SIX

Contact the Institutional Ethics Committee at your university/hospital/Area Health Service.

**a** Find out what the core composition of an Institutional Ethics Committee is as determined by the NHMRC.

**b** What is the composition of the Institutional Ethics Committee at your university/hospital/Area Health Service?

## ACTIVITY SEVEN

Using the elements of a consent form (Box 6.3) that are appropriate, and the example provided on page 158 of the textbook, develop a consent form that could be used in the study by Kermode (1995) in Appendix C.

## ACTIVITY EIGHT



It is 1942 and you are the first doctorally prepared nurse at your hospital. You are approached by Sister Kenney to show the doctors that her treatment for spasms (that is, paralysis of poliomyelitis) is the right way to treat patients. How would you respond to her? What would be your ethical concerns related to this research? Note: A summary of Sister Kenney's methods and ideas follows.

It may be helpful to read the article describing Kenney's life and ideas by Oppewal in *Image: Journal of Nursing Scholarship* 29: 83–7, 1997. (All references cited below can be found in this article.)

*By age 23, Elizabeth was an established bush nurse. She delivered babies and cared for the sick … in 1911, she encountered a young girl in constant pain, muscular pain that increased severely when touched. The child's legs were contracted in twisted positions, and her back and neck were misaligned. Confused by this condition, Nurse Elizabeth telegrammed Dr McDonnell for advice. The return message stated: Infantile paralysis. No known treatment. Do the best you can with the symptoms presenting themselves (Kenney & Ostenso, 1943; Morris, 1972; Oppewal, 1997).*

*Relying on keen observation, caring concern and past knowledge from studying human anatomy, Elizabeth experimented to relieve the child's pain. She had never read or heard of a medical treatment for infantile paralysis, or poliomyelitis, as it was later called. Fearful that contractures and deformities would permanently result unless the child's muscles relaxed, she tried applying heated salt placed in a bag and a linseed meal poultice. Both were too heavy. However, the child did respond to heat from a wool blanket torn into strips then placed in boiling water and wrung dry. Upon awakening from a relaxed sleep, the child said, 'I want them rags that wells my legs!'*

*A year elapsed before Elizabeth discussed this first, and five other cases with Dr McDonnell. He was surprised to learn that none of her patients developed deformities. The orthodox medical treatment at that time was to immobilise the affected limbs during the painful period. Deformity resulted when the healthy muscle in a muscle pair pulled the affected muscle out of shape. Unfortunately, many polio victims treated with immobilisation sustained some type of crippling. Elizabeth explained that she successfully treated spasms with moist heat …*

*Although many patients who were treated with the Kenney method achieved relief and did not develop deformities, her methods were not endorsed by the medical community in Australia. Instead, she was ridiculed by the medical community and accused of being politically motivated. After the death of her main supporter, Dr McDonnell, who had stated: 'She has knocked our theories into a cocked hat, but her treatment works, and that's all that counts'; she decided to bring her ideas to the United States (Kenney & Ostenso, 1943).*

*Following her arrival in America, Kenney again received little support from the medical community. Even though Sister Kenney understood the importance of obtaining medical sanction, she recognised the revolutionary nature of her method … To avoid being labelled a quack Sister Kenney realised that her method had to receive scientific validation (Levine, 1954). Yet, she vacillated between a mission of research and one of instruction. For example, she stated, 'I came to America to teach my method – not to enter a research experiment' (Potter, 1941).*



*Kenney realised that American physicians wanted systematic proof that her empirically demonstrated method worked. But performing a valid experiment on the Kenney method of immobilisation raised ethical problems. No parents would allow their children to receive a treatment that was not the most effective that medicine could offer (Kenney & Ostenso, 1943; Potter, 1941).*

**a** What is your response to Kenney?

**b** What is the major ethical issue involved in the design of this study?

**c** How would you design a research study to determine the most effective treatment for spasms in poliomyelitis?

## POST-TEST

1 Why is it more difficult to maintain confidentiality in qualitative research studies?

2 If you agreed to collect data for a researcher who had not asked the patient's permission to participate in the research study, which of the patient's rights would you be violating?

3 How would you assess the risk/benefit ratio of the study by Waldenström and Nilsson (1994) in Appendix B of the textbook?

4 Unlike humans, animals cannot give informed consent to participate in a research study. How can their rights be protected?

# 7 Introduction to Design

The term 'research design' is used to describe the overall plan of a particular study. The design is the researcher's approach to answering specific research questions in the most accurate, efficient and feasible way possible. The design ties together the present research problem, the knowledge of the past, and the implications for the future. Thus the choice of design reflects the researcher's experience, expertise, knowledge and biases.

## Learning outcomes

On completion of this chapter the student should be able to do the following:

- identify the major components of a research design
- identify threats to internal validity
- identify threats to external validity
- describe the relationship between the research design and internal and external validity
- critically analyse the strengths and limitations of the chosen design for specific studies.

## ACTIVITY ONE

Match the definition of the terms in Column A with the research design terms in Column B. Each term is used no more than once and not all terms will be used.

### COLUMN A

- **a** A plan for conducting a research study
- **b** All parts of a study follow logically from the problem statement
- **c** Methods to keep the study conditions constant during the study
- **d** Consideration as to whether or not the study is possible and practical to conduct
- **e** A sample of subjects with similar characteristics
- **f** Process to ensure every subject has an equal chance of being selected
- **g** Degree to which a research study is consistent within itself
- **h** Degree to which study results can be applied to the larger population

### COLUMN B

- external validity
- internal validity
- accuracy
- design
- control
- random sampling
- feasibility
- homogeneity
- objectivity



## ACTIVITY TWO

For each of the research projects outlined below, identify the type of threat to internal validity from the following list. Explain the reason there is a problem, and suggest how the problem could be corrected.

- history
- instrumentation
- maturation
- mortality
- selection bias
- testing

**a** Nurses on a maternity unit want to study the effect of a new hospital-based teaching program on mothers' confidence in caring for their newborn babies. The researchers mail out a survey one month after discharge.

**b** In a study of the results of a hypertension teaching program conducted at a senior citizens centre, the blood pressures taken by volunteers using their personal equipment were compared before and after the program.

**c** A major increase in cigarette taxes occurs during a one-year follow-up study of the impact of a smoking cessation program.

**d** The smoking cessation rates of an experimental group consisting of volunteers for a smoking cessation program were compared with the results of a control group of persons who wanted to quit on their own without a treatment program.

**e** Thirty per cent of the subjects dropped out of an experimental study of the effect of a job training program on employment of young unemployed women. Over 90 per cent of the drop-outs were women with children, while the majority of subjects successfully completing the program were not parents.

**f** The researcher tested the effectiveness of a new method of teaching drug dosage and solution calculations to nursing students using a standardised calculation exam at the beginning, midpoint and end of a two-week course.

## ACTIVITY THREE

The term 'research design' is an all-encompassing term for the overall plan to answer the research questions, including the method and specific plans to control other factors that could influence the results of the study.

To become acquainted with the major elements in the design of a study, read the study by Waldenström and Nilsson (1994) in Appendix B in the textbook and answer the following questions:

**a** What was the setting for the study?

**b** Who were the subjects?



**c** How was the sample selected?

**d** What information was missing?

**e** Was this a homogenous sample?

**f** How were variables measured and constancy maintained?

**g** Which group served as the control group?

## ACTIVITY FOUR

Use the critiquing criteria in Chapter 7 to critique the research design of the Waldenström and Nilsson (1994) study in Appendix B of the textbook. (Explain your answers.)

**a** Is the design appropriate?

**b** Is the control consistent with the research design?

**c** Does the design used reflect the issues of economy?

**d** Does the design logically flow from the problem, framework, literature review and hypothesis?

**e** What are the potential threats to internal validity?

**f** What are the controls for threats to internal validity?

**g** What are the potential threats to external validity?

**h** What are the controls for threats to external validity?

## ACTIVITY FIVE

Review the Dracup et al. (1997) study in Appendix D of the textbook. Briefly assess the major components of the research design.

**a** What is the purpose of the study?

**b** What is the setting for the study?

**c** Who are the subjects?

**d** How is the sample selected?

**e** How were variables measured?

## POST-TEST

Match the definition of the terms in Column A with the research design terms in Column B. Each term is used no more than once and not all terms will be used.

### COLUMN A

**a** Used to hold steady the conditions of the study

**b** Used to describe that all aspects of a study logically follow from the problem statement

**c** The believability between this study and the world at large

**d** These developmental, biological, or psychological processes operate within a person over time and may influence the results of a study

**e** Time, subject availability, equipment, money, experience and ethics are factors influencing this aspect

**f** Selection bias, mortality, maturation, instrumentation, testing and history influence this aspect of a study

**g** Voluntary, rather than random, assignment to an experimental or control condition creates this situation

### COLUMN B

- consistency
- mortality
- control
- internal validity
- feasibility
- external validity
- selection bias
- accuracy
- reliability
- history
- maturation

# 8 Quantitative Research Design

A researcher chooses the design that allows a given situation or problem to be studied in the most accurate, efficient and feasible way possible. Experimental and quasi-experimental designs allow researchers to test the effects of nursing interventions and infer cause–effect relationships. However, not all problems are able to be studied by these types of design. Non-experimental designs can help to clarify problems and assess relationships between variables. The choice of design is dependent on the development of knowledge relevant to the problem, plus the researcher's experience, expertise, preferences and resources.

## Learning outcomes

On completion of this chapter the student should be able to do the following:

- identify the components of experimental, quasi-experimental and non-experimental designs
- identify the type of quantitative design used in specific studies
- critique the application to clinical practice for various experimental, quasi-experimental and non-experimental studies.

## ACTIVITY ONE

Match the descriptions in Column A with the list of types of experimental and quasi-experimental designs in Column B. Each term is used no more than once and not all terms will be used.

### COLUMN A

**a** Type of design known as one that has two groups identical to the true experimental design plus an experimental after-group and a control after-group

**b** Research approach used when only one group is available to study for trends over a longer period of time

**c** Also known as the post-test only control group design in which neither the experimental group nor the control group is pretested

**d** When a researcher wants to compare results obtained from an experimental group with a control group, but was unable to conduct pretests or to randomly assign subjects to groups

**e** A design with three properties: randomisation, control and manipulation

**f** Subjects are unable to be randomly assigned into experimental and control groups but are able to be pretested and post-tested

### COLUMN B

- true experiment
- Solomon four-group
- after-only experiment
- non-equivalent control group
- after-only non-equivalent control group
- time series
- evaluation research



## ACTIVITY TWO

Review the Waldenström and Nilsson (1994) study in Appendix B of the textbook, then answer the following questions.

**a** The classic experiment has three properties: randomisation, control and manipulation of variables. How were each of these conditions applied in this study?

**b** List the implications of this study for nursing practice.

**c** What difference would there be in interpreting the results if the researcher had not used randomisation?

**d** What difference would there be in interpreting the results if the researcher had not used a control group?

## ACTIVITY THREE

The education department in a large hospital wants to test a program to educate and change nurses' attitudes regarding pain management. They have a questionnaire that measures nurses' knowledge and attitudes about pain. Your responsibility is to design a study to examine the outcome of this intervention program.

**a** You decide to use a Solomon four-group design. Complete the chart below with an X to indicate which of the four groups receive the pretest and post-test pain questionnaire and which receive the experimental teaching program.

| | PRETEST | TEACHING | POST-TEST |
|---|---|---|---|
| Group A | ________ | ________ | ________ |
| Group B | ________ | ________ | ________ |
| Group C | ________ | ________ | ________ |
| Group D | ________ | ________ | ________ |



**b** How would you assign nurses to each of the four groups?

**c** What would you use as a pretest for the groups receiving the pretest?

**d** What is the experimental treatment?

**e** What is the outcome measure for each group?

**f** Based on your reading, for what types of issues is this design particularly effective?

**g** What is the major advantage of this type of design?

**h** What is a disadvantage of this type of design?

## ACTIVITY FOUR

For each of the following descriptions of experimental or quasi-experimental studies, identify the type of design used in the study and the advantages and disadvantages of this design by answering the following questions:

- What type of design was used?
- What are the advantages of this design?
- What are the disadvantages of this design?

**a** *The purpose of this study was to evaluate the relationship of pulmonary rehabilitation to psychosocial adjustment to COPD and use of health care services. Adjustment scores and use of health care services were compared for 13 individuals who had not had formal pulmonary rehabilitation and 17 individuals who had completed a formal pulmonary rehabilitation program (Lewis & Bell, 1995).*

**b** *The effectiveness of a special intervention to help patients decrease dietary fat intake, reduce smoking, and increase exercise was conducted with 138 women who had coronary artery bypass surgery. Subjects were randomly assigned into special intervention or usual care groups. Risk factors and lifestyle behaviors were measured at baseline and 1 year after surgery (Allen, 1996).*

**c** *The performance of 56 students in an accelerated baccalaureate nursing program for college graduates and a traditional baccalaureate nursing program were compared. Students in each group completed the pretest and the posttest on nursing performance (McDonald, 1995).*

**d** *The purpose of the study was to compare behavioral and interactional differences in irritable and nonirritable infants. Forty infants and their mothers were assessed every 3 weeks from 4 weeks to 16 weeks of age (Keefe et al., 1996).*

## ACTIVITY FIVE

Identify whether the following studies are experimental or quasi-experimental. Use the abbreviations from the key provided, and include reasons for your answer.

***Key***

E Experimental

Q Quasi-experimental

**a** Fifty teenage mothers are randomly assigned into an experimental parenting support group and a regular support group. Before the program and at the end of the three-month program, mother–child interaction patterns are compared between the two groups.



**b** Patients on two separate units are given a patient satisfaction with care questionnaire to complete at the end of their first hospital day and on the day of discharge. The patients on one unit receive care directed by a nurse case manager, and the patients on the other unit receive care from the usual rotation of nurses. Patient satisfaction scores are compared.

**c** Students are randomly assigned to two groups. One group receives an experimental independent study program and the other receives the usual classroom instruction. Both groups receive the same post-test to evaluate learning.

**d** A study was conducted to compare the effectiveness of a music relaxation program with silent relaxation on lowering blood pressure ratings. Subjects were randomly assigned into groups and blood pressures were measured before, during and immediately after the relaxation exercises.

## ACTIVITY SIX

Determine an answer for each of the following items. Some terms will be used more than once. Once you have an answer, study the diagram to find each answer. The words will always be in a straight line. They may be read up or down, left to right, right to left, or diagonally. When you find one of the words, draw a circle around it. Any single letter may be used in more than one word.

| | | | | | | | | | | | | | | |
|---|---|---|---|---|---|---|---|---|---|---|---|---|---|---|
| L | O | N | G | I | T | U | D | I | N | A | L | D | M | E |
| C | I | S | P | U | E | Q | W | H | X | O | I | Y | H | X |
| C | R | F | L | G | Y | Q | E | R | C | X | E | C | G | P |
| U | W | O | L | Z | S | B | Q | F | H | V | O | H | H | O |
| N | T | L | S | C | I | S | Z | A | R | R | O | I | U | S |
| L | G | T | R | S | D | L | D | U | R | Z | L | D | O | T |
| U | E | I | O | I | S | Q | S | E | D | L | Y | W | O | F |
| I | U | W | S | J | J | E | L | O | S | Y | U | H | I | A |
| G | T | D | K | X | O | A | C | I | E | M | D | I | I | C |
| Q | W | R | E | E | T | O | K | T | T | E | S | T | A | T |
| A | S | A | M | I | K | E | N | B | I | B | H | U | L | O |
| D | U | O | O | K | L | H | N | P | H | O | B | Z | V | F |
| M | C | N | G | U | L | U | E | O | L | Y | N | R | K | C |
| K | A | M | F | G | U | P | Q | S | B | Z | L | A | H | T |
| L | W | J | F | V | N | E | W | J | S | W | L | E | L | Y |



**a** This type is better known for breadth of data collected than depth.

**b** A major disadvantage is the length of time needed for data collection.

**c** The main question is whether or not variables co-vary.

**d** This word means after the fact.

**e** This eliminates the confounding variable of maturation.

**f** This quantifies the magnitude and direction of a relationship.

**g** Collects data from the same group at several points in time.

**h** Can be surprisingly accurate if the sample is representative.

**i** Uses data from one point in time.

**j** This is based on two or more naturally occurring groups with different conditions of the presumed independent variable.

## ACTIVITY SEVEN

Listed below are a series of advantages and disadvantages for various types of non-experimental designs. For each type of design pick from the list at least one advantage (A) and one disadvantage (D) that accurately describes a quality of the design. Then insert the A or D and the appropriate number in the list following.

**ADVANTAGES**

A1 A great deal of information can be economically obtained from a large population.

A2 Ability to assess changes in the variables of interest over time.

A3 Explores relationship between variables that are not inherently able to be manipulated.

A4 Offers a higher level of control than a correlational study.

A5 They facilitate intelligent decision making by using objective criteria to guide process.

A6 Each subject is followed separately and serves as his/her own control.

A7 Stronger than retrospective studies because of the degree of control on extraneous variables.

**DISADVANTAGES**

D1 The inability to draw a causal linkage between two variables.

D2 An alternative hypothesis could be the reason for the relationships.

D3 The researcher is unable to manipulate the variables of interest.

D4 The researcher is unable to determine a causal relationship between variables because of lack of manipulation, control and randomisation.

D5 The information obtained tends to be superficial.

D6 The researcher must know sampling techniques, questionnaire construction, interviewing and data analysis.

D7 No randomisation in sampling because studying pre-existing groups.

D8 Internal validity threats, such as testing and mortality, are present.



**a** Correlation studies

**b** Cross-sectional

**c** Descriptive/exploratory

**d** Ex post facto

**e** Longitudinal

**f** Prediction studies

**g** Prospective

**h** Retrospective

**i** Survey

## ACTIVITY EIGHT

Each of the following are excerpts from non-experimental studies. For each example, determine the type of design used from the list provided. Not all designs are used as examples, and designs may be used more than once. Note, some studies use more than one type of non-experimental design.

***Key***

| | |
|---|---|
| C | Correlation studies |
| CS | Cross-sectional |
| D/E/S | Descriptive/exploratory/survey studies |
| E | Ex post facto |
| L | Longitudinal |
| M | Methodological |
| MA | Meta-analysis |
| PS | Prediction studies |
| P | Prospective |
| R | Retrospective |

**a** *Historical evidence shows women's attempts to achieve the current societally mandated esthetic ideals. Although a sociocultural impact is generally acknowledged, no measurement instrument has been developed to empirically confirm it. A questionnaire measuring the respondent's recognition and acceptance of the prevailing societal message was developed and validated in a series of 3 studies (Heinberg et al., 1995).*

**b** *[The objective of Sherman's 1996 study was to] use Rogers' (1992) framework of the science of unitary human beings to examine relationships among spirituality, perceived social support, death anxiety, and nurses' willingness to care for AIDS patients. The data collection instruments used were: Spiritual Orientation Inventory, the Personal Resource Questionnaire-85, the Templer Death Anxiety Scale, and the Willingness to Care for AIDS Patients Instrument. The findings: Willingness to care for AIDS patients was positively correlated with spirituality and perceived social support, and negatively correlated with death anxiety (Sherman, 1996).*

**c** *A computerised Clinical Information System (CIS) used for the majority of patient charting and medical records was installed … in the intensive care unit (ICU) of a large Australian hospital … A survey was issued to all nursing staff of the ICU to identify factors that affected attitudes towards computers in the critical care environment. Factors resulting in negative attitudes could then be targeted through training and support for users. The study showed that nursing experience had a statistically significant effect on motivation to use computers. A strong relationship was evident between the concepts of beliefs, attitudes, and motivation (Marasovic et al., 1997).*

**d** *Critical care services are an identified resource intensive component of health care provision. Examining cost containment and clinical effectiveness in this speciality is therefore highly appropriate, although difficult to achieve in practice. The studies reviewed in this paper utilised various methodologies to capture different components of service and patient costs. The methods included combinations of per diem costs, hospital charges, direct consumption, and unspecified cost estimates. Medical fees were commonly excluded, and other costs such as equipment and overheads were often not identified. Some more recent studies used clinical costing methods to* *capture individual patient-specific data, and demonstrated the feasibility and importance of these projects. Differing methods and data collection resulted in a limited comparative analysis, but issues requiring further research are highlighted (Elliott, 1997).*

**e** *The purpose of this study was to examine the health behaviors of nursing students as they entered and again as they completed their baccalaureate nursing education to see what lifestyle changes occurred as students were exposed to a healthcare curriculum. The procedure followed was that of the Health Promoting Lifestyle Profile, a 48-item instrument administered to students during the first and again during the last semester of their nursing program (Riordan & Washburn, 1997).*

**f** *[The purpose was] ... to survey paternal worries, concerns, stresses, or problems and the type of support received by men whose partners were prescribed bed rest at home, or in the hospital or both ... A national subsample of 59 men whose mates had been on pregnancy bed rest were randomly selected in 1995 from a non-random select sample of individuals who had contacted a bed-rest support group (Sidelines) for information. The mean total length of bed rest was 92.1 days ... The majority of the women were on both home and hospital bed rest (36%), while 21 were solely on home bed rest, and two were only on hospital bed rest; 53% had been on bed rest within the last year and all but 17% had been on bed rest within the last 2 years ... (Maloni & Ponder, 1997).*

**g** *This empirical study explored the attitudes and participation of registered nurses (RNs) in New South Wales (NSW), Australia in continuing professional education ... A 25-item questionnaire was developed and mailed to a random sample of 500 RNs currently licensed to practice within NSW. Respondent anonymity was assured by having the Nurses Registration Board generate the random sample and undertake the mailing (Kersaitis, 1997).*



## POST-TEST

Identify the type of experimental or quasi-experimental design for each of the following examples. Use the numbers from the key provided.

### *Key*

**1** After-only experimental

**2** After-only non-equivalent control group

**3** True experiment

**4** Non-equivalent control group

**5** Solomon four-group

**a** Nurses are randomly assigned to a new self-study program or the usual ECG teaching program. Knowledge of ECGs is tested before and after the program for both groups.

**b** Babies who tested positive on toxicology screening at birth are randomly assigned into groups to either receive routine care or to receive a special public health nurse intervention program. Health outcomes are tested and compared at six months.

**c** A school nurse clinic is set up at one school. Health care outcomes are measured at the end of a year from that school and compared with health outcomes at a comparable school that does not have a clinic.

**d** Diabetic patients were randomly assigned to either one of two control groups receiving routine home health care or to one of two groups with a new diabetic teaching program. Patients in one of the control groups and in one of the teaching groups took a test of diabetic knowledge as soon as they were assigned to a group. Patients in the other two groups were not pretested. All patients completed a post-test at the conclusion of the three-week program.

**e** A new peer AIDS prevention program was implemented in one high school. A second high school without the program served as a control group. An AIDS knowledge test was administered at both schools before and after the program was completed.

# 9 Qualitative Approaches to Research: Methods and Sampling

Qualitative research continues to gain recognition as a sound method for investigating the complex human phenomena less easily explored using quantitative methods. Empirical studies are essential for investigating particular variables, but are less helpful in understanding human responses and life experiences. Nurse researchers and investigators from other disciplines are discovering the increased value of findings obtained through qualitative studies. Nurses can be better prepared to critique the appropriateness of a research design and identify the usefulness of the study findings when the differences between quantitative and qualitative research designs are understood.

Chapters 9 and 13 of the textbook are specifically devoted to the qualitative method of research and focus on four commonly used approaches. Chapter 9 includes research elements of each approach as they relate to 'Identifying the phenomenon' and 'Structuring the study'. Chapter 13 deals with the remaining elements of data collection, analysis and interpretation.

## Learning outcomes

On completion of this chapter the student should be able to do the following:

- distinguish the characteristics of qualitative research from those of quantitative research
- recognise the uses of qualitative research
- identify the qualitative approaches of phenomenological, grounded theory, ethnographic and historical methods
- identify the key aspects of 'Identifying the phenomenon' and 'Structuring the study' as they relate to the four commonly used qualitative methods
- evaluate a qualitative research report using critiquing criteria.

## ACTIVITY ONE

The reasons for selecting a qualitative design rather than a quantitative one are based on the research question and the purpose of the study. Recognition of the differences between qualitative research and quantitative research enables the nurse to better interpret the research report findings and identify ways they might be applied.

For each of the following research characteristics write the term qualitative or quantitative as appropriate.

**a** Humans are a composite of many body systems that can be objectively measured.

**b** Truth is the subjective expression of reality as perceived by the subject.

**c** Data collection is complete when saturation is reached.

**d** A clear context-free picture is the aim of the study.

**e** Life context is the matrix of human-human-environment relationships.

**f** Large numbers of subjects are extensively studied.

**g** Extraneous variables need to be eliminated.

**h** The researcher goes where the data lead.

**i** The whole is greater than the sum of the parts.



## ACTIVITY TWO

Match the terms in Column A with the appropriate definitions in Column B.

### COLUMN A

**a** Information becomes repetitive

**b** Select experiences to test ideas

**c** Outsider's view

**d** Identify personal biases about phenomenon

**e** Insider's view

**f** Symbolic categories

**g** Individuals willing to teach investigator about the phenomenon

**h** In-depth description of phenomenon

**i** Provide another perspective of phenomenon

**j** Inductive approach to develop theory about social processes

### COLUMN B

- theoretical sampling
- emic view
- etic view
- data saturation
- secondary sources
- bracketed
- case study method
- grounded theory method
- domains
- key informants

## ACTIVITY THREE

**a** Four qualitative research methods are discussed in the textbook in terms of the research elements: identifying the phenomenon and structuring the study (which includes three components):

- Identifying the phenomenon
- Structuring the study
  - the research question
  - the researcher's perspective
  - sample selection.

Under each research element, briefly describe a key aspect that relates to each of the four qualitative methods: phenomenology, grounded theory, ethnography, historical.

**b** Explain how the author(s) 'identify the phenomenon' in the studies by:

- Barclay et al. (1996) in Appendix A of the textbook
- Kermode (1995) in Appendix C of the textbook.

## ACTIVITY FOUR

The literature review usually provides a background for understanding a research problem. However, not all qualitative research methods follow the traditional approach to literature reviews.

Read the study by Barclay et al. (1996) in Appendix A in the textbook.

**a** Identify the main theme of the literature review.

**b** Explain two ways in which the literature in this study could be applied to nursing practice.

**c** Comment on the authors' use of the literature.

## ACTIVITY FIVE

Four qualitative methods of research are the phenomenological, grounded theory, ethnographic and historical methods.

For each characteristic listed below, indicate which method of qualitative research it describes. There may be more than one correct answer. Use the abbreviations from the key provided.

***Key***

A Phenomenological

B Grounded theory

C Ethnographic

D Historical

**a** Uses primary and secondary sources.

**b** Uses 'emic' and 'etic' views of subjects' worlds.

**c** Research questions are action or change oriented.

**d** Central meanings arise from subjects' descriptions of lived experience.

**e** Truth is a lived experience.

**f** Uses theoretical sampling to analyse data.

**g** Discovers 'domains' to analyse data.

**h** Provides insight on the past and serves as a guide to the present and future.

**i** Establishes fact, probability or possibility.

**j** States individuals' history is a dimension of the present.

**k** Attempts to discover underlying social forces that shape human behaviour.

**l** Interviews 'key informants'.

**m** Presents data as a synthesised chronicle.

**n** Focuses on describing cultural groups.

**o** Establishes reliability through external and internal criticism.

**p** Researcher 'brackets' personal bias or perspective.

**q** Subjects are currently experiencing a circumstance.



**r** Collects remembered information from subjects.

**s** Involves 'field work'.

**t** Describes events from the past.

**u** May use photographs to describe current behavioural practices.

**v** Uses symbolic interaction as a theoretical base.

**w** Uses an inductive approach to understanding basic social processes.

## ACTIVITY SIX

Review the paper by Kermode (1995) in Appendix C and complete the following questions.

**a** What was the qualitative method used in the research study?

- phenomenological
- grounded theory
- ethnographic
- historical

**b** What was the main focus of the study?

- patients with AIDS
- the experience of living with AIDS

- nursing practice
- nurses' knowledge and understanding

**c** What were sample size and selection based upon?

- data saturation and personal experience of the phenomenon
- random selection
- advisement of key informants
- convenience sampling

## ACTIVITY SEVEN

Based on the four methods of qualitative research described in the textbook:

**a** Select the method you found the most interesting.

**b** Explain the things you find especially appealing about this method.

**c** List three subject areas in which this method might be helpful in developing nursing knowledge.

**d** Choose one of these subject areas and identify a research question to be studied.

**e** Describe the perspective you would adopt as the researcher.

**f** Identify the characteristics of the study subjects, where you will locate them, how many subjects you might include, and why.



## POST-TEST

**1** What qualitative research method would be most appropriate for studying the impact of culture on the birthing experience?

**a** phenomenological

**b** grounded theory

**c** ethnographic

**d** historical

**2** What qualitative research method would be most appropriate for answering the question: 'What factors influenced the move of nursing education to the tertiary sector?'

**a** phenomenological

**b** grounded theory

**c** ethnographic

**d** historical

**3** The qualitative method that uses symbolic interaction as the theoretical base for research is known as which of the following?

**a** phenomenological

**b** grounded theory

**c** ethnographic

**d** historical

**4** What is the qualitative method that attempts to construct the meaning of human experience through dialogue?

**a** phenomenological

**b** grounded theory

**c** ethnographic

**d** historical

**5** Why are hypotheses not appropriate in qualitative studies?

**6** What is the basic underlying philosophy of qualitative inquiry? How does it differ from that of quantitative inquiry?

# 10 Sampling

Sampling consists of choosing the elements to be used in answering the research question. The ideal sampling strategy is one in which the elements truly represent the population of interest while controlling any bias. Considerations of efficiency, practicality, ethics and availability of subjects frequently alter the ideal sampling strategy for a given study.

## Learning outcomes

On completion of this chapter the student should be able to do the following:

- discuss the advantages and disadvantages of various probability and non-probability sampling strategies
- identify the sampling strategy used in study examples
- evaluate the congruence between the sample used and the population of interest
- critique the sampling component of specific studies.

## ACTIVITY ONE

Identify the category of sampling for each of the following sampling strategies. Use the abbreviations from the key provided.

***Key***

P Probability sampling

N Non-probability sampling

**a** Simple random sampling

**b** Purposive sampling

**c** Cluster sampling

**d** Quota sampling

**e** Convenience sampling

**f** Systematic sampling

**g** Stratified random sampling

## ACTIVITY TWO

For each of the examples of studies given below, identify the sampling strategy used from the following list. Check the glossary in the textbook for definition of terms.

- convenience sampling
- quota sampling
- purposive sampling
- simple random sampling
- stratified random sampling
- cluster sampling
- systematic sampling

**a** The sample for the study of critical thinking behaviour of undergraduate Bachelor of Nursing students consisted of students enrolled in first year and third year in three schools of nursing. In each program, students were invited to participate until a total sample representing 10 per cent of first year students and 10 per cent of third year students was obtained.

**b** Every eighth person on the diabetic clinic patient roster was asked to participate in the study. A table of random numbers was used to select the beginning of the sampling within the first sampling interval.

**c** Using a table of random numbers, the sample consisting of fifty subjects was selected from the list of all mothers giving birth in New Zealand during the first six months of the year.

**d** The sample was selected from residents of six nursing homes in Adelaide and consisted of cognitively impaired persons with no physical impairments or other psychiatric illnesses.

**e** To select the sample, twenty-five rehabilitation centres were randomly selected from the list of all rehabilitation centres in Australia. Ten nurses were randomly selected from each site for a final sample of 250 nurses.

**f** The sample consisted of twenty chronic pain patients participating in a multi-modal pain management program.

**g** To study educational opportunities for nurses from various ethnic groups, a list of all nurses in Victoria was sorted by ethnicity. The sample consisted of 10 per cent of the nurses in each ethnic group, selected according to a table of random numbers.

## ACTIVITY THREE

Refer to the study by Waldenström and Nilsson (1994) in Appendix B of your textbook.

**a** Was the sample adequately described? Yes No

**b** Do the sample characteristics correspond to the larger population? Yes No Partially

**c** Is this a probability or non-probability sample?

**d** Is the sample size appropriate? Yes No Unsure

## ACTIVITY FOUR

Using the critical thinking decision path in the textbook (page 279), indicate whether or not the following statements are true or false.

**a** Non-probability sampling is associated with less generalisability to the larger population.

**b** Convenience sampling followed by random assignment into treatment groups increases generalisability.

**c** Non-probability sampling strategies are more time consuming than probability strategies.

**d** Random sampling has the greatest risk of bias and is moderately representative.

**e** The advantage of ease of sampling is associated with the greatest risk of bias and limited representativeness of the sample.

**f** Purposive sampling produces the least generalisable sample of the sampling strategies listed.

## ACTIVITY FIVE

Review the study by Dracup et al. (1997) in Appendix D of the textbook. Using the critiquing criteria listed in Chapter 10 of the textbook (page 285), critique the sampling process used in this study.

## POST-TEST

Complete the following sentences.

1 Sampling strategies are grouped into two categories: ________________ sampling and ________________ sampling.

2 ________________ sampling is the use of the most readily accessible persons or objects as subjects in a study.

3 Advantages of ________________ sampling are low bias and maximal representativeness, but the disadvantage is the resource use in drawing a sample.

4 A(n) ________________ can be used to select an unbiased sample or unbiased assignment of subjects to treatment groups.

5 A(n) ________________ sample is one whose key characteristics closely approximate those of the population.

6 ________________ criteria are used to select the sample from all possible units and ________________ may be used to restrict the population to a homogeneous group of subjects.

7 Types of non-probability sampling include ________________, ________________ and ________________ sampling.

8 Successive random sampling of units that progress from large to small and meet sample eligibility criteria is known as ________________ sampling.

9 In certain qualitative studies, subjects are added to the sample *until* ________________ occurs (new data no longer emerge during data collection).

10 A statistical technique known as ________________ may be used to determine sample size in quantitative studies.

# 11 Data Collection Methods

*Observe, probe*
*Details unfold*
*Let nature's secrets*
*Be stammeringly retold*

*Goethe*

As a consumer of research the reader needs the skills to evaluate and critique data collection methods in published research studies. In order to achieve these skills it is helpful to have an appreciation of the process or the critical thinking 'journey' the researcher has taken. Each of the preceding chapters covered important preliminary steps in the research planning and design phases prior to data collection. Although most researchers are eager to begin data collection, the planning is very important. It includes identifying and prioritising data needs, developing or selecting appropriate data collection tools, and selecting and training data collection personnel before proceeding with the actual collection of data.

The five types of data collection methods differ in their basic approach and the strengths and weaknesses of their characteristics. Readers should be prepared to ask questions about the appropriateness of the measures chosen by the researcher to gather data about the variable of concern. This includes determining the objectivity, consistency, quantifiability, observer intervention and/or obtrusiveness of the chosen data collection method.

## Learning outcomes

On completion of this chapter the student should be able to do the following:

- describe the five types of data collection methods used in nursing research
- describe the advantages and disadvantages of selected data collection methods
- match types of variables to the most appropriate data collection method
- critique data collection components of the methodology of specific studies
- evaluate the applicability of published research studies based upon a critique of the data collection method
- discuss the role of data collection in the overall research process.

## ACTIVITY ONE

Review each of the articles referenced below (Appendices A–D of the textbook), paying particular attention to the sections that relate to data collection methods. Answer the questions in relation to what you understand from the article. For some questions there may be more than one answer.

### *Barclay et al. (1996)*

**a** Which data collection method was used in this research study?

- a physiological measure
- an observational measure
- an interview measure
- a questionnaire measure
- records or available data

**b** Comment on the appropriateness of the data collection method.

**c** In grounded theory studies the concepts emerge from the data, therefore the questions should be:

- tape recorded
- open-ended
- close-ended
- time-limited.



**d** What is the significance of meeting the requirements of within-group homogeneity when conducting gender specific focus groups?

### *Waldenström and Nilsson (1994)*

**a** Which data collection method was used in this research study?

- a physiological measure
- an observational measure
- an interview measure
- a questionnaire measure
- records or available data

**b** Comment on the appropriateness of the data collection method.

**c** Critically review the data collection process.

**d** Which items on the questionnaire(s) have been identified as data collected using a Likert-type scale?

### *Kermode (1995)*

**a** What data collection method was used in this research study?

- a physiological measure
- an observational measure

- an interview measure
- a questionnaire measure
- records or available data

**b** Comment on the appropriateness of the data collection method.

**c** Explain the purpose of the follow-up interviews in this study.

**d** Differentiate between structured, semi-structured and unstructured interviews.

### *Dracup et al. (1997)*

**a** What data collection method was used in this research study?

- a physiological measure
- an observational measure
- an interview measure
- a questionnaire measure
- records or available data

**b** Comment on the data collection procedures.

**c** What were the variables studied in this research?

**d** The vast majority of subjects in this study (96 per cent) preferred the researchers to read out the questions rather than completing the questionnaire themselves. How does this affect the data collection process?



## ACTIVITY TWO

Using the content of Chapter 11 in the textbook complete the following word search exercise. Answer the questions and find the word in the puzzle.

**a** Methods that use technical instruments to collect data about patient's physical, chemical, microbiological or anatomical status.

**b** The distortion of data as a result of the observer's presence.

**c** Best used when a large response rate and an unbiased sample is necessary.

**d** Using this data collection method can be subject to problems of availability, authenticity and accuracy.

**e** An especially useful strategy when there are a finite number of questions to be asked and they are clear and specific.

**f** Appropriateness and two other concepts are essential when critiquing the data collection methods.

**g** Not used much in nursing because it raises too many ethical issues, especially those related to informed consent.

**h** The consistency of observations between two or more observers.

**i** The process of translating concepts/variables into measurable phenomena.

**j** A scale that uses close-ended items with a fixed number of alternative responses.

**k** The method for objective, systematic and quantitative description of communications and documentary evidence.

**l** Following the construction of a new instrument it is necessary to do this with a group of people who are similar to the target population.

| | | | | | | | | | | | | | | | | | | | | | | |
|---|---|---|---|---|---|---|---|---|---|---|---|---|---|---|---|---|---|---|---|---|---|---|
| D | E | L | I | V | E | R | S | T | A | T | I | S | T | I | C | S | Y | E | S | P | I | S |
| S | S | A | C | A | B | I | N | E | T | F | O | R | K | A | Z | O | S | P | E | I | N | Z |
| I | A | W | O | P | E | R | A | T | I | O | N | A | L | I | S | A | T | I | O | N | T | T |
| G | T | S | N | O | R | N | E | V | E | R | B | Y | D | N | E | A | U | X | B | J | E | O |
| N | S | Y | S | T | E | M | A | T | I | C | A | J | H | T | B | S | T | V | S | E | R | I |
| I | F | L | I | K | E | R | T | V | E | S | O | B | E | R | R | O | Y | A | E | R | R | L |
| F | A | K | S | C | A | L | E | S | N | O | V | N | O | C | A | A | U | L | R | R | A | L |
| H | C | U | T | A | C | R | A | T | I | M | A | P | V | E | T | P | U | I | V | A | T | Y |
| Y | T | B | E | B | H | I | R | T | E | M | A | H | V | K | K | I | C | D | A | T | E | M |
| P | C | O | N | T | E | N | T | A | N | A | L | Y | S | I | S | P | V | O | T | E | R | E |
| R | O | Y | C | B | K | D | S | I | S | R | T | S | A | D | V | A | N | I | I | R | R | T |
| E | R | E | Y | A | D | U | G | K | A | T | P | I | B | I | O | I | O | G | T | R | E | 1 |
| A | V | S | I | B | R | Q | U | E | S | T | I | O | N | N | A | I | R | E | N | Y | L | W |
| C | I | A | R | E | S | E | A | R | C | H | L | L | R | E | A | C | E | S | O | L | I | I |
| T | O | B | M | E | X | C | E | L | A | E | O | O | D | A | T | A | C | O | V | I | A | S |
| I | U | E | A | E | V | A | L | I | D | S | T | G | N | O | S | T | O | O | E | A | B | H |
| V | N | Y | E | S | S | I | N | T | E | R | V | I | E | W | S | A | R | F | R | B | I | E |
| I | H | A | P | P | I | E | N | E | S | S | P | C | A | T | A | G | D | U | N | I | L | L |
| T | X | C | I | T | E | D | E | L | P | H | I | A | T | O | T | P | S | N | V | V | I | L |
| Y | A | B | L | E | A | C | O | N | C | E | A | L | M | E | N | T | O | O | T | T | T | I |
| A | I | K | E | V | A | L | I | K | E | I | I | A | V | C | O | N | S | U | M | Y | Y | E |

## ACTIVITY THREE

You are reviewing a study and concealment is necessary; in other words, there is no other way to collect the data and the data collected are unlikely to have negative consequences for the subject.

**a** Give a specific example of what kind of study this could be.

**b** How would you obtain subjects' consent?

**c** What is this process called?

## ACTIVITY FOUR

You are asked to participate in discussions about impending research in your community. The purpose of the study is to identify the health status, beliefs, practices and preventive services currently known and used, and accessibility/availability of health service needs for the residents of your rural community.

Outline your critical thinking journey by describing what you would consider in the selection of a data collection method. Review each method and discuss the pros and cons for choosing a specific method. State the rationale for your final selection. What would be your thinking about instruments and types?

## ACTIVITY FIVE

Using the content of Chapter 11 in the textbook, choose the correct response for each question. Some questions may have more than one correct answer.

**a** What is a primary advantage of physiological measurement as a data collection instrument?

- The measuring tool never affects the phenomena that are being measured
- It is one of the easiest types of methods to implement
- It is unlikely that study participants/subjects can distort the physiological information
- The instrument has objectivity, sensitivity and precision
- All of the above

**b** What is the process of translating concepts that are of interest to the researcher into observable and measurable phenomena called?

- Objectivism
- Systematisation
- Subjectivism
- Operationalisation

**c** Which of the following would be considered as disadvantages of using observational data collection methods?

- Individual bias may interfere with the data collection
- Ethical concerns may be increasingly significant to researchers using observational data collection methods
- Individual judgements and values may influence the perceptions of the observers
- All of the above

**d** What is collection of data from each subject in the same or in a similar manner known as?

- Repetition

- Dualism
- Consistency
- Recidivism

**e** What is consistency of observations between two or more observers known as?

- Intra-rater reliability
- Inter-rater reliability
- Consistency reliability
- Repetitive reliability

**f** In nursing research, when might questionnaires be used as an appropriate method of data collection?

- Whenever expense is a concern for the researcher
- When a researcher is interested in obtaining information directly from the subjects
- When the researcher needs to collect data from a large group of subjects that are not easily accessible
- When accuracy is of the utmost importance to the researcher

**g** Which of the following would be considered as advantages of using existing records or available data to answer a research question?

- The use of available data reduces the risk of researcher bias in data collection
- Time involvement in the research study can be reduced by the use of available records or data
- Consistent collection of information over periods of time allows the researcher to study trends
- All of the above

**h** Which of the following is not consistent with a Likert scale?

- It contains close-ended items
- It contains open-ended items
- It contains lists of statements
- It evaluates items on the amount of agreement

**i** A researcher wants to use a questionnaire in a study but cannot find one that will gather the information required about a particular variable. The decision is made to develop a new instrument. Which of the following should the researcher do?

- Define the construct, formulate the items, and assess the items for content validity
- Develop instructions for users and pilot the instrument
- Estimate reliability and validity
- All of the above

## POST-TEST

Read each question thoroughly and then circle the correct answer. For some questions more than one answer may be correct.

1 Answering research questions pertaining to psycho-social variables can best be done by using which data gathering technique(s)?

- **a** Observation
- **b** Interviews
- **c** Questionnaires
- **d** All of the above

2 Physiological and biological measurement might be used by nurse researchers when studying which of these variables?

- **a** A comparison of student nurses' first year results and their Year 12 scores
- **b** Hypertensive clients' responses to a stress test
- **c** Children's dietary patterns
- **d** The degree of pain relief achieved following guided imagery

3 Scientific observations should fulfil which of the following conditions?

- **a** Observations are consistent with the study objectives
- **b** Observations are standardised and systematically recorded
- **c** Observations are checked and controlled
- **d** All of the above

4 In a research study, a participant observer spent regularly scheduled hours in a homeless shelter and occasionally stayed overnight. The people staying in the home were told that this person was conducting a research study. The researcher freely engaged in conversation and openly observed the homeless. What is the observational role of the researcher?

- **a** Concealment without intervention
- **b** Concealment with intervention
- **c** No concealment without intervention
- **d** No concealment with intervention

5 In unstructured observation, which of the following might occur?

- **a** Recording of extensive field notes
- **b** Informing subjects what behaviours are being observed
- **c** Frequent recording by the researcher of interesting anecdotes
- **d** All of the above

6 Self-report measures are usually more useful than observation measures in obtaining information about which of the following?

a Socially unacceptable or private behaviours

b Complex research situations when it is difficult to separate processes and interactions

c When the researcher is interested in character traits

d All of the above

7 In order to evaluate the adequacy of various data collection methods, which of the following should be observed in the written research report?

a Clear identification of the rationale for selecting a physiological measure

b The problems of bias and reactivity addressed with observational measures

c A clear explanation of how interviews were conducted and how interviewers were trained

d All of the above

8 Although it is acceptable to use multiple instruments within a research study, the study is more acceptable if only one method is used for the data collection.

a True

b False



9 Social desirability is seldom a concern for researchers when the data collection method used in the study is interviews.

a True

b False

10 The researcher who invests significant amounts of time in the development of an instrument has a professional responsibility to publish the results.

a True

b False

11 In conducting a research study, the researcher has a responsibility to ensure that all study subjects received the same information and data were collected from all participants in the same manner.

a True

b False

# 12 Reliability and Validity in Quantitative Research

The reliability and validity of data collection instruments must be sound in order to create confidence in the results of a study. A research consumer must be able to critique the reliability and validity of instruments giving particular consideration to the possibility of systematic and random error in a study.

## Learning outcomes

On completion of this chapter the student should be able to do the following:

- understand the differences between systematic and random error
- discuss reliability and validity as they relate to data collection instruments
- compare content, criterion and construct validity in the selection of the instrument used in research
- define the various forms of reliability – stability, homogeneity and equivalence
- critique the reliability and validity reported in specific studies.

## ACTIVITY ONE

Either random error (R) or systemic error (S) may occur in a research study. For each of the following examples, identify the type of measurement error and how the error might be corrected.

**a** The scale used to obtain daily weights was inaccurate by 500 grams less than actual weight.

**b** Students chose the socially acceptable responses on an instrument to assess attitudes towards AIDS patients.

**c** Confusion existed among the evaluators on how to score the wound healing.

**d** The subjects were nervous about taking the psychological tests.

## ACTIVITY TWO

Validity is concerned with whether or not the measurement tools are actually measuring what they are supposed to measure. Match the definitions in Column A with a term or method in Column B.

Consult the glossary in the textbook to check definition of terms.

### COLUMN A

**a** The three major kinds of validity

**b** A researcher used this to establish content validity of a new rating scale for maternal attachment

**c** This kind of validity was assessed by correlating scores of the Learned Helplessness Scale with the Beck Hopelessness Scale and Rosenberg Self-Esteem Scale (Flynn, 1997)

**d** In the same study, Flynn (1997) used Radloff's Center for Epidemiologic Studies Depression Scale (CES-D). This kind of validity was found through factor analyses that consistently supported the four theoretical categories of the instrument

**e** The use of a variety of measurement strategies to assess convergent and divergent validity

**f** This kind of validity is an intuitive, preliminary type of instrument evaluation

### COLUMN B

- concurrent validity
- face validity
- content validity
- factor analysis
- contrasted groups
- hypothesis testing
- construct validity
- multi-trait–multi-method approach
- convergent
- predictive validity
- criterion validity
- rating from a panel of experts
- divergent

**COLUMN A**

**g** Two ways of measuring construct validity, an assessment of the theory underlying the instrument

**h** The kind of validity expected with an instrument that measured a construct similar to coping

**i** The kind of validity expected with an instrument that measured a construct opposite to coping

## ACTIVITY THREE

An instrument is considered reliable if it is accurate and consistent. If the concept being studied is stable, the same results should occur when measurement is repeated.

**a** Name three concepts related to reliability.

**b** Give an example of each of the two types of tests for stability.

**c** In what instance would it be better to use an alternative form rather than a test–retest measure for stability?



## ACTIVITY FOUR

Homogeneity is a measure of internal consistency. All items on the instrument should be complementary and measure the same characteristic or concepts. For each of the examples given below, identify which of the following tests for homogeneity is described:

- item-total correlation
- split-half reliability
- Kuder-Richardson (KR-20) coefficient
- Cronbach's alpha

**a** The odd items of the test have a high correlation with the even numbers of the test.

**b** Each item on the test using a 5-point Likert scale had a moderate correlation with every other item on the test.

**c** Each item on the test ranged in correlation from 0.62 to 0.89 with the total.

**d** Each item on the true–false test had a moderate correlation with every other item on the test.

## ACTIVITY FIVE

In a study by Daniels et al. (1995), the collection of blood for BSL determination by a variety of nurses was assessed. What is this assessment of the data collectors called?

## ACTIVITY SIX

In this activity use the critiquing criteria listed in Chapter 12 of the textbook (pages 336–7) to evaluate the instruments used in the study by Good (1995), reprinted in Chapter 18 of the textbook. Refer to the section discussing the measures (pages 455–6) to answer the following questions.

**a** Internal consistency coefficients for the State Trait Anxiety Inventory (STAI) were 0.89 for pre-operative anxiety and 0.90 for post-ambulatory anxiety of pain. Is this adequate for reliability?

**b** A correlation of r = 0.37 was demonstrated between the two measurement times – pre-operative and post-ambulation. What is your interpretation of the reasons for this figure?

**c** Was reliability established for the Distress of Pain Scale?

## POST-TEST

Using the following terms, complete the sentences for the type of validity or reliability discussed. Terms may be used more than once.

- content validity
- test–retest reliability
- factor analysis
- Cronbach's alpha
- convergent validity
- alternate or parallel form
- divergent validity
- inter-rater reliability

**1** In tests for reliability the self-efficacy scale had a(n) _____________ of 0.88, demonstrating internal consistency for the new measure.

**2** The ABC social support scale demonstrated _______________ validity with correlation of 0.84 with the XYZ interpersonal relationships scale.

**3** _________ validity was supported with a correlation of 0.42 between the ABC social support scale and the QRS loneliness scale.

**4** The investigator established __________________ validity through evaluation of the cardiac recovery scale by a panel of cardiac clinical nurse specialists. All items were rated 0 to 5 for importance to recovery and only items scoring above an average of 3 were kept in the final scale.

**5** The results of the ________________ were that all the items clustered around three factors, lending support to the notion that there are three dimensions of coping.

**6** The observations were rated by three experts. The ________________ reliability among the observers was 94 per cent.

**7** To assess _______________ reliability, subjects completed the locus of control questionnaire at the beginning of the project and two weeks later. The correlation of 0.86 supports the stability of the concept.

**8** Bennett et al. (1996) developed an instrument: the Cardiac Event Threat Questionnaire (CTQ). They established _______________ validity by reviewing the literature, reviewing concerns identified by patients recovering from a cardiac event, and had the items critiqued by a panel of experts.

**9** The results of the CTQ that measured threat were highly correlated with the results of a test measuring negative emotions. This established _______________ validity.

**10** Bennett et al. (1996) reported that internal consistency reliabilities of the five factors of the CTQ were computed with the _________________ statistic.

# 13 Qualitative Approaches to Research: Data Collection, Analysis and Interpretation

Chapter 9 of this text provides activities which apply to the research elements of 'identifying the phenomenon' and 'structuring the study' as they relate to the four commonly used methods of qualitative research. This chapter provides activities which illustrate the way in which data collection procedures, data analysis and interpretation are used and presented in qualitative research studies. These elements continue the qualitative research process resulting in the narrative summary of the researcher's attempts to capture the human experience that is the focus of the study.

Conducting a scientifically rigorous study is essential for all researchers. However, the achievement of such rigour differs between qualitative and quantitative research. For those who undertake qualitative research it is necessary to make explicit how they established and maintained the rigour which is specific to this type of inquiry.

## Learning outcomes

On completion of this chapter the student should be able to do the following:

- identify the key aspects of data collection, analysis and interpretation as they relate to the four commonly used qualitative methods
- use existing articles to identify the elements of data collection, analysis and interpretation
- recognise the processes used in establishing methodological/scientific rigour in qualitative research
- reconcile the use of both qualitative and quantitative research in the same study.

## ACTIVITY ONE

Four qualitative research methods – phenomenology, grounded theory, ethnography and historical – are discussed in the textbook in terms of the research elements: (a) data collection, (b) data analysis and (c) data interpretation (describing the findings).

Briefly describe a key aspect of each research element as it relates to each of the four qualitative methods.

## ACTIVITY TWO

Review Kermode (1995) in Appendix C of the textbook and complete the following multiple choice items.

**a** What was the data gathering process?

- Observation and structured interview guide
- Semi-structured interviews
- Focus groups
- Participant observation

**b** What methods were used for data analysis?

- Synthesis of essences
- Constant-comparative method
- Identification of themes
- Open coding of categories

**c** The findings of the study were described by using:

- the steps in the process and the logic of the method
- a narrative elaboration of experiences
- an integration of field notes and interviews
- a well-synthesised chronicle approach.



## ACTIVITY THREE

**a** How do researchers establish scientific rigour in a qualitative study?

**b** Differentiate the ways in which the two qualitative studies in the textbook (Appendices A and C) established methodological/scientific rigour.

## ACTIVITY FOUR

Describe what you understand by the term 'triangulation'.

## ACTIVITY FIVE

Refer back to your answers for Activity seven in Chapter 9 and using the same subject area and research question:

**a** Describe the data collection method(s) you would use for this study.

**b** Briefly explain an important aspect of data analysis using the method you have chosen.

**c** Describe what factors you would consider when describing the findings.

**d** Describe how you might use the knowledge gained from this study in nursing practice.

## POST-TEST

**1** To what does the term 'saturation' in qualitative research refer?

- **a** Data repetition
- **b** Subject exhaustion
- **c** Researcher exhaustion
- **d** Sample size

**2** In qualitative research, data are often collected by which of the following?

- **a** Questionnaires sent out to subjects
- **b** Observations of subjects in their natural settings
- **c** Interviews
- **d** All are correct

**3** What is meant by the term 'researcher as instrument'?

**4** What are the five basic elements of qualitative research methodology?

**5** What does the 'constant-comparative' method of analysis mean?

**6** What are the advantages of using data triangulation in a research study?

**7** Discuss the strengths and weaknesses of the phenomenological method of inquiry in terms of data collection and analysis techniques.

# 14 Descriptive Data Analysis

The activities in this chapter focus on the concept of measurement and the use of descriptive statistics. Descriptive statistics are used to describe sample characteristics. Some studies rely on descriptive statistics as the major data analysis strategy, while other studies use a combination of descriptive and inferential statistics.

## Learning outcomes

On completion of this chapter the student should be able to do the following:

- distinguish between the four levels of measurement in datasets
- interpret measures of central tendency and variation
- evaluate the use of descriptive statistics in specific studies.

## ACTIVITY ONE

Match the level of measurement found in Column B with the appropriate example(s) in Column A. The levels of measurement in Column B will be used more than once.

| COLUMN A | COLUMN B |
|---|---|
| **a** Amount of emesis | N Nominal |
| **b** Height or weight | O Ordinal |
| **c** High, moderate, low level of social support | I Interval |
| **d** Satisfaction with nursing care | R Ratio |
| **e** Use or non-use of contraception | |
| **f** Amount of empathy | |
| **g** Number of metres walked | |
| **h** Type A or Type B behaviour | |
| **i** Body temperature measured with Celsius thermometer | |

## ACTIVITY TWO



Read the following excerpts from specific studies. Identify the variable (or variables) and indicate what level of measurement would apply.

**a** *Mood state was defined as the client's full range of feelings about participation in the drug trial and was measured using the Bipolar Form of the Profile of Mood States. The four-point Likert-type Scale contained 72 items measuring mood over the previous week (Wineman et al., 1996).*

**b** *Perceived health status of the subjects was determined by asking them to choose one statement indicating their current state of physical health. Choices ranged from 1, indicating that 'I think my present health is very good' to 5, indicating 'I think my present health is very poor' (Johnson, 1996).*

**c** *Diet diaries were kept for 3 days (2 weekdays and 1 weekend day). Each subject's dietary intake of carbohydrate, protein, and fat was used to calculate total calories and calories from each nutrient group … (Lipp, Deane & Trimble, 1996).*

**d** *Data were obtained from local health department records and birth certificate data … Information gathered from the nursing and WIC records included: Mother's age at delivery … trimester of initial contact with client … infant birthweight … (Baldwin & Chen, 1996).*

## ACTIVITY THREE

Review your answer for Activity Two excerpt **a** and refer to Table 1 below.

**a** What is the variable of interest in this table? What part of Table 1 requires your attention?

**b** Name the types of statistics used to describe the information about mood state.

**c** What level of measurement is needed to use these statistics?

**d** Does the level of measurement named in your answer to question **c** match the level of measurement you indicated in your answer for Activity Two, excerpt **a**?

**Table 1 Means, Standard Deviations and Ranges for Study Scales**

| SCALES | MEAN | STANDARD DEVIATION | STUDY RANGE | POSSIBLE RANGE |
|---|---|---|---|---|
| Mood state | 40.7 | 36.65 | –41 to 123 | –197 to 233 |
| Hopefulness | 184.7 | 26.14 | 108 to 237 | 48 to 240 |
| Illness uncertainty | 77.3 | 10.07 | 57 to 106 | 27 to 135 |
| Perceived stress | 23.1 | 25.39 | 0 to 92 | 0 to 100 |
| Coping effectiveness | 159.3 | 77.20 | 0 to 326 | 0 to 360 |
| N = 59 | | | | |

*Source: Wineman et al., 1996*

## ACTIVITY FOUR

Refer to your answer for Activity Two, excerpt **c**.

**a** Are the data in Table 2 below reported using the appropriate descriptive statistics for the level of measurement? Explain your answer.

**b** Write a narrative interpretation of the data in the first line of Table 2. Include any additional information you know about this study.



**Table 2 Diet Diary**

| | MEAN | RANGE | SD |
|---|---|---|---|
| Total calories/day | 3322 | 435–7753 | 1263 |
| Total grams fat/day | 132 | 17–334 | 58.3 |
| % total calories/day in fat | 34 | 18–48 | 5.2 |
| Total mg sodium/day | 5369 | 840–9999 | 2189 |
| N = 78 | | | |

*Source: Lipp, Deane, Trimble, 1996*

## ACTIVITY FIVE

Review Table 1 of the Sharts-Hopko et al. (1996) article, reprinted in the textbook on page 474, and answer the following questions.

**a** How many total subjects participated in the study?

**b** Assuming a normal distribution, what would be the age range for 95 per cent of the sample?

**c** What proportion of subjects were not African American?

**d** Write a narrative description of the sample.

**e** What are your thoughts on the sample distribution? (Hint: Consider the standard deviation scores.)

**f** How could this variance be assessed?

## ACTIVITY SIX

Table 3 following is reproduced from a research study by Goodwin (1997). The study was designed to describe the association among several measures of the marital relationship and the health of the wife with chronic fatigue and immune dysfunction syndrome (CFIDS). Study the information in the table and then answer the questions that follow.

**Table 3 Means, Standard Deviations and Paired t-tests for Husbands' and Wives' Scores**

| SCALES | HUSBANDS M(SD) | WIVES M(SD) | n | t |
|---|---|---|---|---|
| **Marital variables** | | | | |
| Marital adjustment | 110.63 (18.13) | 110.15 (17.74) | 127 | .36 |
| Marital empathy | | | | |
| Spouse ability | 45.21 (14.44) | 46.20 (15.68) | 114 | –.66 |
| Self ability | 32.66 (7.83) | 33.58 (6.32) | 115 | –1.17 |
| Marital support | 52.66 (7.80) | 53.22 (9.87) | 130 | –.71 |
| Marital conflict | 28.59 (8.43) | 27.65 (9.50) | 127 | 1.10 |
| **CFIDS symptoms** | | | | |
| Number of symptoms | 42.97 (11.86) | 46.73 (8.28) | 128 | –3.82*** |
| Mean problem score | 2.83 (0.69) | 3.03 (0.58) | 128 | –3.40** |
| Total problem score | 121.16 (44.16) | 142.63 (39.30) | 128 | –6.80*** |

*p<.05 **p<.01 ***p<.001; 2 tailed

Note: CFIDS = chronic fatigue and immune dysfunction syndrome

Source: Goodwin, 1997



**a** What is the highest mean reported?

**b** For what group and what variable is the highest mean reported?

**c** Which measure of the marital variables is the most homogeneous (that is has the least variation)?

**d** Which group (that is husbands or wives) was the most heterogeneous in reporting CFIDS symptoms?

**e** The following is the text in which the researchers discuss the data in Table 3. (Note: Ignore the p<.01, p< .001 and p<.001 notation.)

*No significant differences were found in the couples' reported marital relationship variables of marital adjustment, marital empathy, marital support and marital conflict. The paired wives and husbands' descriptions of the wives' CFIDS symptoms were significantly different. Wives and husbands' reported number of symptoms … the mean problem scores … and the total problem scores … were significantly different (Goodwin, 1997).*

Does the information in the table and textbook agree?

## ACTIVITY SEVEN

Two outpatient clinics measured client waiting time as one indicator of effectiveness. The mean and standard deviation of waiting time in minutes is reported below. Which outpatient clinic would you prefer, assuming that all other things are equal? Explain your answer.

| | CLINIC 1 | CLINIC 2 |
|---|---|---|
| Mean (in minutes) | 40 | 25 |
| Standard deviation (in minutes) | 10 | 45 |

## ACTIVITY EIGHT

This is a reverse crossword puzzle; that is, the puzzle is already completed. Identify the appropriate clue for each answer of the puzzle.

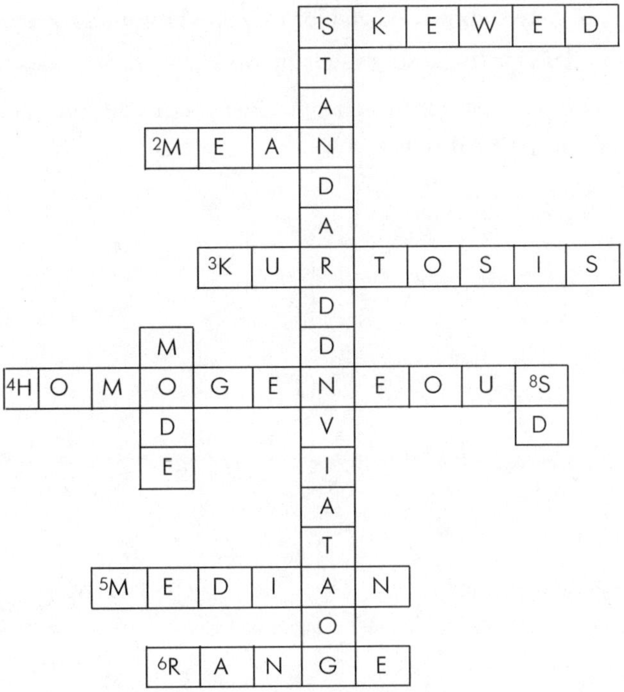


### *Clues*

**a** Measure of central tendency used with interval and ratio data

**b** Measure of variation that shows the lowest and highest number in a dataset

**c** Marks the score where 50 per cent of the scores are higher and 50 per cent are lower.

**d** Describes a distribution characterised by the presence of a tail

**e** Abbreviation for standard deviation

**f** Sixty-eight per cent of the values in a normal distribution fall between ±1 of this statistic

**g** The value that occurs most in a dataset

**h** A dataset with a standard deviation of 3 is more ________ than a dataset with a standard deviation of 12

**i** An asymmetrical dataset

## ACTIVITY NINE

Using the studies in Appendices A–D in the textbook, answer the following questions regarding the use of descriptive statistics in each study. You may wish to refer to the critical thinking path (see page 368 of the textbook) and the critiquing criteria in Chapter 14 (see page 381 of the textbook).

**a** Was the use of descriptive statistics appropriate for this type of study?

**b** Were descriptive statistics used in the study?

**c** What data were summarised and/or explained through the use of descriptive statistics?

**d** Were the descriptive statistics used appropriately?

There is no post-test for this chapter. Please consider the critical thinking challenges on page 384 of the textbook.

15

# Inferential Data Analysis

Descriptive statistics are valuable for summarising data and enabling examination of the salient features about a group of data, but clinicians often require more data about whether or not an intervention under investigation has enough evidence to substantiate application to clinical practice. The use of inferential statistics allows inferences to be drawn about subjects in a study being equivalent to a larger patient population.

## Learning outcomes

On completion of this chapter the student should be able to do the following:

- understand the link between specific research aims and appropriate inferential tests
- interpret the results of specific inferential statistical tests
- critique the use of inferential statistics in specific studies.

## ACTIVITY ONE

Review the introductory and method sections of the Good (1995) paper, reprinted on pages 452–458 of the textbook, to answer the following questions.

**a** What were the research hypotheses tested in this study?

**b** What were the independent and dependent variables?

**c** At what level of measurement were the variables measured?

**d** Were the inferential statistical tests appropriate?

## ACTIVITY TWO

Review the Waldenström and Nilsson (1994) study in Appendix B of the textbook to answer the following questions.

**a** What was the basic question addressed by Waldenström and Nilsson (1994)?

**b** Is the research hypothesis written or implied?

Data in Table 1 (reprinted on page 544 of the textbook) compares the experimental and control groups for a number of variables.

**c** What is the appropriate statistical test for the variables: parity, civil status and ethnic background? Explain your answer.



**d** Why were t-tests used for the variables: age, length of gestation and years of education?

In Table 2 (reprinted on page 545 of the textbook), differences between the two groups are displayed.

**e** What is your interpretation of the first line of the table: 'Antenatal education, %'?

**f** What statistical test would have been used to test differences in length of post-partum stay?

## ACTIVITY THREE

Review Table 3 of the paper by Sharts-Hopko et al. (1996) reprinted on page 476 of the textbook and then answer the following questions.

**a** What do the negative values mean?

**b** Explain, in your own words, the statistically significant relationships highlighted in the table for perceived self-efficacy (PSE).

**c** Explain the meaning of '$p<.001$'.

## ACTIVITY FOUR

Refer to the Dracup et al. (1997) study in Appendix D of the textbook and then answer the following questions.

**a** What was the basic question addressed by the researchers?

**b** What were the socio-demographic variables identified by the researchers which were significantly associated with delay in seeking treatment?

**c** What socio-demographic variables were found to be not significantly associated with delay in treatment?

**d** Following further analysis from the researchers, what were determined as the five independent predictors of delay?

There is no post-test for this chapter. Please consider the critical thinking challenges on page 405 of the textbook.

# 16 Analysis of the Findings

The last sections of a research report, the results and conclusion sections, answer the question 'So what?'. It is in these two sections that the investigator 'makes sense' of the research, critically synthesises the data, ties them to a theoretical framework, and builds on a body of knowledge. The two sections are very important because they describe the generalisability of the findings and offer recommendations for further research. Well-written, clear and concise results and conclusion sections provide valuable information for nursing practice. Conversely, poorly written results and conclusion sections leave a reader bewildered, confused and wondering how or if the findings are relevant to nursing.

## Learning outcomes

On completion of this chapter, the student should be able to do the following:

- know the difference between the results sections of a study and the discussion sections of a study
- interpret table and figure findings from a research report
- describe the various generalisations and limitations of a research report
- synthesise data and identify implications for nursing
- identify recommendations from a research report.

## ACTIVITY ONE

Read the results (findings) and discussion sections of the study by Waldenström and Nilsson (1994) in Appendix B of the textbook then answer the following questions.

**a** The randomisation into two groups produced a significant difference between the experimental and control groups in terms of the number of pregnancies (parity). True False

**b** When the women in the control group (CG) were compared to those in the experimental group (EG), the latter had less pharmacological pain relief and were discharged earlier. True False

**c** At two months after birth there was a 9.3 per cent difference in breast feeding between the two groups. True False

**d** The control group needed significantly more sedation during labour than the experimental group. True False

**e** Of the initial 617 women in the experimental group, 33 per cent were either transferred or withdrew from the study. True False

**f** According to the findings there was a strong relationship between being in the birth centre group and the variables of 'sore nipples' and 'milk stasis'. True False

## ACTIVITY TWO



Discuss the implications for practice from the results of the Waldenström and Nilsson (1994) study. Assume you are a midwife in charge of an antenatal clinic and a first time mother (and her partner), who is keen to breast feed, asks your advice about where to give birth. Outline what you would say and give reasons for your advice.

## ACTIVITY THREE

Interpret the following statistical findings from the Waldenström and Nilsson (1994) study.

**a** When comparing the experimental and control groups in terms of the mean length of post-partum days, a statistic of $p = <0.001$ was found. Explain what this means.

**b** At two months 58 per cent of women in the experimental group and 56 per cent of women in the control group had used a breast pump at least once, revealing a statistic of 95 per cent CI = -4.0-9.1, $p = 0.44$. What conclusion may be reached from this finding?

**c** How did the researchers compare the two groups in terms of the level of support provided by the midwife during labour, and what does the result mean?

## ACTIVITY FOUR

The following statistical components are used in the Waldenström and Nilsson (1994) article. Match them with the correct terms.

| COLUMN A | COLUMN B |
|---|---|
| **a** multiple regression | • sample size |
| **b** $p = <0.001$ | • student's t-test |
| **c** $n = 617$ | • probability level |
| **d** $t =$ | • measure of relationship between one interval level dependent variable and several independent variables |

## ACTIVITY FIVE

When probability level is calculated as $p<0.05$ and the researcher has previously set the alpha level of significance at 0.05 the researcher must reject the null hypothesis and accept the alternate hypothesis. True False

## ACTIVITY SIX

The interpretation of qualitative research results and conclusions differs significantly from that of quantitative research findings. After reading the article by Barclay et al. (1996) in Appendix A of the textbook, complete the following.

**a** Explain what is meant by an 'audit trail' and how the researchers used it in their analysis of men's experiences.

**b** Comment on the way in which the authors used the subjects' narrative in the results section of the article.

**c** What is the significance of confusion as a category finding?

**d** The researchers identified a conceptual model based on the relationships between the core and other categories found in the analysis of data obtained from the subjects. Briefly explain your interpretation of the model.

**e** After reading the results and discussion sections of the article, list three implications for the practice of midwifery.

**f** Provide two to three suggestions for further research based on the findings from this study.

## ACTIVITY SEVEN

Being able to interpret tables in research articles is an important part of the critiquing process. Dracup et al. (1997) studied the concept of delay in seeking treatment after the onset of symptoms of myocardial infarction, and the factors contributing to the delay. Read their article in Appendix D of the textbook and then answer the following questions. Refer to Box 1 in the article

**a** Explain the difference between the columns of mean hours, median hours and interquartile range (H).

**b** Note which level of education was associated with a significantly longer delay in seeking treatment.

**c** Comment on the relationship between a person's level of income and their response to cardiac symptoms.

**d** Identify the two errors in column 1 (Patient Characteristics).

Dracup (1997) et al. placed more emphasis than previous researchers on the social/cognitive factors that might influence response time to cardiac symptoms.
Refer to Box 2

**a** Which variable(s) were the least significant in regard to response to cardiac symptoms?

**b** What percentage of respondents were concerned about troubling others when they experienced cardiac symptoms?

**c** What was the relationship between the most significant social/cognitive factors and response time to cardiac symptoms?

**d** What are the implications for future nursing research based on the results of the findings presented?

Different patient characteristics and perceptions have an influence on delay in seeking treatment after the onset of cardiac symptoms.
Refer to Box 3

**a** Differentiate the odds ratio results for 'symptoms seen as not serious' and the 'symptom of dizziness'.

**b** Comment on the relationship between patients who experience intermittent symptoms and the time taken to seek treatment.

**c** Comment on which one of the variables in Box 3 was identified as the most important factor in predicting delay in seeking treatment for cardiac symptoms and whether or not it is amenable to nursing intervention.

**d** What is the alpha level of significance set by the researchers for the study?

## ACTIVITY EIGHT

After reading the results and discussion sections of the Dracup et al. (1997) article, identify three implications for nursing practice.

## ACTIVITY NINE

Kermode (1995) explored Patients' Experiences of Nursing Interventions During Hospitalisation with an AIDS-defining Illness. Read Appendix C of the textbook and then complete the following questions.

**a** What was the purpose of the study?

**b** What comments can you make about the author's description of the way in which the data were analysed?

**c** Table 1 refers to the AIDS-related themes that were identified from the data. What comments have you got to make about the way in which the themes were addressed in the textual representation of the data?

**d** How did the works of Benner, and Benner and Wrubel help to inform the data analysis and interpretation?

**e** Comment on the way in which the data have been used to exemplify the theme of nursing interventions through the categories of Care and Carelessness.

**f** Critically review the section in the article titled Implications for Nursing Practice.

## POST-TEST

**1** When a research hypothesis is supported through testing, it may be assumed that the hypothesis was which of the following?

**a** proved

**b** accepted

**c** rejected

**d** disconfirmed

**2** Limitations of a study describe its weaknesses. True False

**3** The results section of a research study includes all the following except:

**a** hypothesis testing results

**b** tables and figures

**c** statistical test description

**d** limitations of the study.

**4** Unsupported hypotheses mean that the study is of little value in generating knowledge. True False

**5** Tables in research reports should meet all the following criteria except:

**a** being clear and concise

**b** restating the text narrative

**c** economising the text

**d** summarising the text narrative.

**6** The discussion section provides an opportunity for the investigator to do all of the following except:

**a** describe implications from the research results

**b** relate the results to the literature review

**c** make generalisations to large populations of subjects

**d** suggest areas for further research.

**7** Hypothesis testing is described in the discussion section of the research report. True False

# 17 Evaluating the Qualitative Research Report

Read through the study and the written critique that is part of Chapter 17 in the textbook. Following these steps will help you produce a critique of this quality.

1 Read the research report from beginning to end. Do not stop to query particular content or sections. Simply start at the beginning and read to the end. This will give you an impression of the article as a whole.
2 Read through the critiquing guidelines found in Table 17.1 of the textbook.
3 Read the article again and make a note of any thoughts, issues or ideas that occur while reading. The margins of a copy of the journal article are easy places to note anything that needs to be reviewed.
4 Now go through the article section by section. Read the questions from Table 17.1, then read the relevant section of the research report and answer the questions. This material will become the working draft of the written critique.
5 Develop the draft by writing the critique in a narrative style. Appropriate use of language is important. Avoid being heartless or brutal, but raise questions where necessary.

## Learning outcomes

On completion of this chapter the student should be able to do the following:

- identify the influence of stylistic considerations on the presentation of a qualitative research report
- identify the criteria for critiquing a qualitative research report
- evaluate the strengths and weaknesses of a qualitative research report
- describe the applicability of a qualitative research report.

## ACTIVITY ONE

The methods of presentation in qualitative research reports are different from those in quantitative studies. Authors of qualitative research reports are challenged to present the richness of the data within the restrictions of publication guidelines.

Review the article by Barclay et al. (1996) in Appendix A of the textbook to examine the way the researchers presented their data.

In the results section of the article the authors identified six categories that arose from the analysis of their data. Each category is presented and includes example quotes from the data to highlight or exemplify the authors' interpretation. Examine this section of the article and choose one example of the participants' quotes that most accurately reflects the category for you.

**a** anxiety

**b** ambivalence

**c** adjustment

**d** separation

**e** need to know

**f** development

## ACTIVITY TWO



The findings of qualitative studies describe or explain a phenomenon within a specific context. The findings are usually not generalisable to other groups, which means that people who want to apply the findings to others have the responsibility to validate whether they are applicable in a different setting with other groups.

The conceptual model of the relationships between categories in the Barclay et al. (1996) study reveals that for the majority of men confusion dominates their experiences during their partner's first pregnancy. This core category integrates all the other categories except development.

**a** Identify two factors that should be considered if it was intended to apply the findings to other groups of men who are sharing their partner's first pregnancy.

**b** Explain what it means to be 'context bound'.

**c** Could the subject population in the Barclay et al. (1996) study be considered context bound? What are the implications if the study is to be replicated?

**d** Qualitative research is also used to examine important concepts and ideas. How do the findings in the Barclay et al. (1996) study contribute to the existing body of knowledge?

**e** Instrument development is another way that findings from qualitative studies can be used. How might the findings from this study be applied to men who are sharing their partner's first pregnancy?

## ACTIVITY THREE

Critiquing qualitative research enables the nurse to make sense out of a research report, build on the body of knowledge about human phenomena, and consider how knowledge might be applicable to nursing. Learning and applying a critiquing process is the initial step in this direction.

Review Table 17.1 in the textbook and answer the following. Match the activity in Column A with the appropriate term in Column B. Some are used more than once.

**COLUMN A**

**a** The purpose of the study is clearly stated

**b** Semi-structured interviews were used to collect the data

**c** Do the participants recognise the experience as their own?

**d** Purposive sampling was used

**e** Data are clearly reported in the research article

**f** The researcher has remained true to the findings

**g** Recommendations for future research are made

**h** The phenomenon of interest is clearly identified

**i** Participant observation was used ethnographically

**COLUMN B**

- Subject selection
- Study method
- Researcher perspective
- Data analysis
- Application of findings
- Findings described
- Study design



## ACTIVITY FOUR

Locate Table 13.2 in Chapter 13 of the textbook. Use this table to answer the following about the Barclay et al. (1996) study.

**a** Describe what you view as the credibility of the study findings.

**b** Explain what you perceive as the auditability of the findings.

**c** Discuss your perceptions about the fittingness of the findings.

## ACTIVITY FIVE

The Scannell-Desch (1996) article entitled *The Lived Experience of Women Military Nurses in Vietnam During the Vietnam War* (Chapter 17 of the textbook) used phenomenology to study the lived experience of nurses during a war. The participants served from 1965 to 1973 and the majority were volunteers. The data collection for this study was conducted at least twenty years after the war experience. Read this article and think about the design of the study and how you would evaluate the findings.

Using the critiquing guidelines on page 426 of the textbook indicate whether the criteria have been met in the Scannell-Desch (1996) article by responding yes or no to the following:

**a** Statement of the Phenomenon of Interest

**b** Purpose

**c** Method

**d** Sampling

**e** Data Collection

**f** Data Analysis

**g** Credibility

**h** Auditability

**i** Fittingness

**j** Findings

**k** Conclusions, Implications and Recommendations.

## ACTIVITY SIX

Identify at least two concerns about the study discussed in Activity five that you might discuss with the investigator if you had an opportunity.

There is no post-test for this chapter.

# 18 Evaluating Quantitative Research Studies

The activities in this chapter use two articles to give you the opportunity of developing a full critique. See *A Comparison of the Effects of Jaw Relaxation and Music on Post-operative Pain* (Marion Good, 1995) and *Problem-focused Coping in HIV-infected Mothers in Relation to Self-efficacy, Uncertainty, Social Support and Psychological Distress* (Shorts-Hopko et al.) reprinted in the textbook on pages 451–80.

## Learning outcomes

On completion of this chapter the student should be able to do the following:

- describe the criteria for each step of the critiquing process
- evaluate the strengths and weaknesses of a research report
- discuss the implications of the findings of a research report
- construct a critique of a research report.

## ACTIVITY ONE

After reviewing the critiquing guidelines on pages 449–51 of the textbook, read the complete paper by Good (pages 452–63).

**a** While reading the article, consider issues under the following headings:

- Problem statement and purpose
- Review of literature and theoretical framework
- Hypotheses or research questions
- Sample
- Research design
- Methods
- Legal–ethical issues
- Instruments
- Reliability and validity
- Analysis of data
- Conclusions, implications and recommendations.

**b** Write the first draft of a critique.

**c** Compare your statements for each section with the critique provided on pages 464–9.



## ACTIVITY TWO

Read the complete paper by Sharts-Hopko et al. (1996) which is reprinted in the textbook (pages 470–80) and write a critique.

## POST-TEST

Write a full critique of one of the papers in Appendices A–D of the textbook.

# 19 Research Utilisation

Research is important to the clinician as a means to support current practice or to provide data to support a practice change. When using research to support or change practice, the clinician should consider two main aspects. First, what interventions provide the best patient outcomes? If there is no difference in patient outcomes when considering two or more interventions, then cost, in both dollars and time, should also be considered. Second, if there is research support for a practice change, what process should the clinician follow for implementation?

## Learning outcomes

On completion of this chapter the student should be able to do the following:

- interpret a summary table to determine recommendations for practice
- identify organisational forces that affect research utilisation
- evaluate an individual research study for its potential for utilisation in the student's clinical setting.

## ACTIVITY ONE

Table 1 summarises the findings from three studies on the use of heparin versus saline as a flush solution for peripheral intravenous locks of adult patients. Use the table and the additional material following to answer the questions.

**Table 1 Summary Table for Synthesis of Peripheral Lock Flush Solutions**

| | PURPOSE | | VARIABLES AND MEASURES | | | | |
|---|---|---|---|---|---|---|---|
| **Citation** | **Research question** | **Sample size** | **Independent** | **Dependent** | **Statistical test** | **Significance level/results** | **Implications** |
| Geritz (1992) | To compare the efficacy of saline | locks 150 peripheral IV lock sites versus 10 U/mL heparin flush solutions in peripheral IV locks | Saline versus heparin flush in 90 adults | Patency, reasons for solutions | Chi-square t-tests doing lock | p>0.05 No difference in patency or reasons to discontinue lock | Recommended saline as flush maintains same patient outcomes at lower cost |
| Peterson and Kirchhoff (1991) | To compare the efficacy of saline | 20 research studies versus multiple heparin flush solutions in peripheral IV locks | Saline versus heparin flush (1 paediatric, 19 adult) | Patency phlebitis solutions | Meta-analysis of 13 studies that met criteria | d-index values z-scores significance not reached, no difference in phlebitis rates or loss of patency | Small number of paediatric studies, cannot extrapolate to children, did not address cost issues |
| Shoaf and Oliver (1992) | To compare the efficacy of saline versus 10 U/mL heparin flush solutions in peripheral IV | 260 adult surgical patients | Saline versus heparin flush solutions | Patency phlebitis | Randomised blind 2-group design | 95% confidence intervals, no difference in patency or phlebitis | Recommended saline as flushing solution, did not calculate cost differences |

### *Nursing implications and conclusions*

*Based on this study of 260 subjects, there were no significant differences in patency and phlebitis between the use of flushing solutions with normal saline versus a control of 10 U/mL heparin in normal saline injection to maintain an intermittent indwelling intravenous site. The study identified that the use of saline solution alone is less irritating and less expensive. These results support the research of Garrelts et al. (1989); Taylor, Hutchinson, Milliken and Larson (1989); Harrigan (1985); and Epperson (1984).*

*It is recommended that peripheral intermittent intravenous sites are flushed after medication infusions and/or every 8 hours with normal saline solution. As a result of this study and similar findings in other clinical settings, Scott and White Memorial Hospital changed the intermittent intravenous infusion device protocol. Peripheral intermittent infusion devices are now flushed routinely with 1 mL normal saline after drug administration or flushed every 8 hours (Shoaf & Oliver, 1992).*

### Conclusions

*The meta-analysis reveals that there is no significant difference between heparin and saline flush procedures in peripheral intravenous catheters. This finding is supported quantitatively by the low average effect size ($0.076 \pm 0.14$) and by the qualitative research data. Results of all but one study suggest that saline solution as a peripheral intravenous flush solution effectively maintains catheter patency, decreases the complications of heparin, and does not significantly increase the incidence of phlebitis. The discrepant study, however, had serious weaknesses. The lack of difference between the two flush solutions is a positive finding in light of the complications associated with heparin use (Peterson & Kirchhoff, 1991).*

### Discussion

*This study supports the findings of others (Epperson, 1984; Garrelts et al., 1989; Hamilton et al., 1988) that normal saline is as effective as heparin solution in the maintenance of intermittent peripheral venous access devices (Geritz, 1992).*

**a** With the information you have available, does each study meet the criteria for a sound study? Yes No

**b** How do the samples compare in the three studies? Are the patients comparable or different? Are the sample sizes sufficient?

**c** How do the independent and dependent variables in the three studies compare? Are the researchers studying the same variables?

**d** Compare and contrast the results of the three studies. Do they reach the same or different conclusions?

**e** When examining the overall implications of the three studies, do they strongly support a particular flushing solution for peripheral locks? Why or why not? What flush solution do the studies recommend for practice?

**f** If the flush solutions compared in the research studies are equally effective in maintaining patency or peripheral locks, how do they compare in cost according to the authors?



## ACTIVITY TWO

Examine the written protocol on peripheral lock flush solutions and procedures that your ward/unit uses and compare it with what was used in the articles in Activity one. If you use the protocol advocated by the research base, fill in the column for your ward/unit only.

**a** What method of flushing the IV peripheral lock does your ward/unit use?

**b** How does your patient population compare with the samples in the research studies?

**c** Does your ward/unit use the flush solution that the research in Table 1 reports should be used?

**d** If it uses a different peripheral lock flush procedure, how much does your procedure cost, and how much would the saline flush cost in your ward/unit? Use Table 2 to help you with the comparison.

**Table 2 Comparing the Cost of Peripheral Lock Flush Protocols**

| | | SALINE FLUSH PROTOCOL | YOUR PROTOCOL |
|---|---|---|---|
| 1 | Cost of solutions | | |
| | a saline | | |
| | b heparin/hep-saline | | |
| 2 | Number of times solution used at each flush | | |
| | a saline | | |
| | b heparin/hep-saline | | |
| 3 | Cost of saline x number of times used (lines 1a x 2a) | | |
| 4 | Cost of heparin/hep-saline x number of times used (lines 1b x 2b) | | |
| 5 | Total cost of solutions (lines 3 + 4) | | |
| 6 | Minutes of staff time required for flush | | |
| 7 | Average hourly pay | | |
| 8 | Average benefit on-costs (0.20 x line 7 if unsure) | | |
| 9 | Cost of staff time | | |
| | a line 7 + line 8 | | |
| | b line 9a divided by 60 | | |
| | c line 9b x line 6 | | |
| 10 | Cost of flush protocol per flush (lines 5 + line 9c) | | |
| 11 | Number of patients that require a peripheral lock | | |
| 12 | Per cent of peripheral locks that are flushed | | |
| 13 | Total number of peripheral lock flushes (line 11 x line 12) | | |
| 14 | Annual cost of peripheral lock flushes (line 10 x line 13) | | |

- Cost of solution of heparin/hep-saline? Of saline? Single or multi use vials?
- Number of times each solution is used?
- Minutes of staff time required each time the peripheral lock is flushed and average hourly pay (include finding solutions and preparing syringes, as well as administering flush)?
- Cost of staff time required for each peripheral lock flush?
- Number of patients in your ward/unit each day that require a peripheral lock?
- Percentage of patients with a peripheral lock that require flushing the lock?
- Total number of peripheral lock flushes that are administered in your ward/unit each year?
- Difference in annual cost of your ward/unit's protocol and that recommended by the research in the three articles?

## ACTIVITY THREE

Assume that your ward/unit does not use saline flushes for peripheral locks and you would like to change the protocol based on your figures in the preceding activity. After a literature search of additional recently published research you expanded your summary table and have identified a strong research base for the change you are proposing. According to the Stetler/Marram model of research utilisation (Box 19.1 in the text) you have completed Phase II: Validation, and are ready to move to Phase III: Comparative Evaluation. However, you will need to move key people in your ward/unit through Phase II.

**a** In your ward/unit, which individuals and disciplines would it be necessary to convince that the practice change has a sufficient research base?

**b** How will you convince them to accept the evidence that the practice change has strong research support and is applicable to your clinical setting?

**c** If the practice change has comparable patient outcomes to your current practice, how will you demonstrate cost effectiveness, and to whom should you present the evidence?

**d** Once the practice change has been approved, how will you or your ward/unit begin the change process?

**e** After the practice change has been implemented, is there anything else that must be considered?



## ACTIVITY FOUR

Read the Barclay et al. (1996); Waldenström and Nilsson (1994); Kermode (1995); and Dracup et al. (1997) studies found in the appendices in the textbook.

**a** Indicate for each article whether utilisation of the results would be conceptual (C) or decision driven (D).

**b** Think about the implications of each study. Using the questions from Box 19.1 in the text, how important would you consider each study for research utilisation in your clinical setting?

**c** What is the topic's priority for nursing in your setting?

**d** What is the magnitude of the problem in your setting? Does it affect a few or many clinical areas? Each study may be considered a priority if the problem addressed is high frequency, high risk or high cost.

**e** Would the practice change affect length of stay, costs or patient satisfaction?

**f** For each study, if there were a strong research base, would your setting be ready to change, or are there sensitive issues to consider and address?

**g** Is there a research base of other studies on each topic? Look through research indexes to identify other studies on one of the four topics.

There is no post-test for this chapter. Please consider the critical thinking challenges on page 520 of the text.

# References


Allen JK: Coronary risk factor modification in women after coronary artery bypass surgery, *Nurs Res* 45:260–265, 1996.

Baldwin KA, Chen SC: Use of public health nursing services: relationship to adequacy of prenatal care and infant outcome, *Public Health Nurs* 13:13–20, 1996.

Barclay L, Donovan J, Genovese A: Men's experiences during their partner's first pregnancy: a grounded theory analysis, *Aust J Adv Nurs* 13(3):12–24, 1996.

Beck C et al.: Improving dressing behavior in cognitively impaired nursing home residents, *Nurs Res* 46(3):126–132, 1997.

Bennett SJ et al.: Development of an instrument to measure threat related to cardiac events, *Nurs Res* 45:266–270, 1996.

Bloom K, Trice L: The efficacy of individualized computerized testing in nurse education, *Computer Nurs* 15: 82–88:1997.

Bolla CD et al.: Social support as a road map and vehicle: an analysis of data from focus group interviews with a group of African American women, *Public Health Nurs* 13(5):331–336, 1996.

Burns L, Adams L: Alcohol – history taking by nurses and doctors – how accurate are they really? *J Adv Nurs* 25:509–513, 1997.

Daniels G, Poroch D, De Roach J: Bloodletting for BSL: the effects of timing and sites on blood volume, *Aust J Advanced Nurs* 12(3):11–14, 1995.

Dracup K, McKinley S, Moser D: Australian patients' delay in response to heart attack symptoms, *Med J Aust* 166:233–236, 1997.

Elliott D: Costing intensive care services: a review of methods, results and limitations, *Aust Crit Care* 10:55–63, 1997.

Flynn L: The health practices of homeless women: a causal model, *Nurs Res* 46(2):72–77, 1997.

Geritz MA: Saline versus heparin in intermittent infuser patency maintenance ... including commentary by Hoare K and Jensen L with author response, *West J Nurs Res* 14(2):131–141, 1992.

Goodwin SS: The marital relationship and health in women with chronic fatigue and immune dysfunction syndrome: views of wives and husbands, *Nurs Res* 46(3): 138–146, 1997.

Heinberg LJ, Thompson JK, Storner S: Development and validation of the socio-cultural attitudes towards appearance questionnaire, *Inter J Eat Dis* 17:81–89, 1995.

Hoffart N, Woods CQ: Elements of nursing practice model, *Nurs Res* 46(2):72–77, 1997.

Hopp LJ et al.: Incremental threshold loading in patients with chronic obstructive pulmonary disease, *Nurs Res* 45(4):196–202, 1996.

Jackson MS, Schmierer CL, Schneider Z: Development, refinement and future usage of the scale: attitudes toward learning in pregnancy, *Int J Nur Stud* 33:36–46, 1996.

Johnson LE: Social support and physical health in the rural elderly, *Appl Nurs Res* 9:61–66, 1996.

Kang SY, Magura S, Shapiro JL: Correlates of cocaine/crack use among inner city incarcerated adolescents, *Am J Drug Alcohol Abuse* 20:413–429, 1994.

Keefe MR et al.: A longitudinal comparison of irritable and nonirritable infants, *Nurs Res* 45:4–9, 1996.

Kendra MA: Perception of risk by home health care administrators and field workers, *Public Health Nurs* 13(6):386–393, 1996.

Kermode M: Patients' experiences of nursing interventions during hospitalisation with an AIDS-defining illness, *Aust J Advanced Nurs* 12(3):20–30, 1995.

Kersaitis C: Attitudes and participation of registered nurses in continuing professional education in New South Wales, Australia, *J Contin Educ Nurs* 28:135–139, 1997.

Lewis D, Bell SK: Pulmonary rehabilitation, psychosocial adjustment, and use of healthcare services, *Rehab Nurs* 20:102–107, 1995.

Lipp EJ, Deane D, Trimble N: Cardiovascular disease risks in adolescent males, *Appl Nurs Res* 9:102–107, 1996.

Maloni JA, Ponder MB: Father's experience of their partners' antepartum bed rest, *Image: J Nurs Schol* 29:183–188, 1997.

Manderino MA, Berkey N: Verbal abuse of staff nurses by physicians, *J Prof Nurs* 13(1):48–55, 1997.

Marasovic C et al.: Attitudes of Australian nurses toward the implementation of a clinical information system, *Comp Nurs* 15:91–98, 1997.

McDonald WK: Comparison of performance of students in an accelerated baccalaureate nursing program for college graduates and a traditional nursing program, *J Nurs Educ* 34:123–127, 1995.

Milligan RA, Flenniken PM, Pugh LC: Positioning intervention to minimize fatigue in breast-feeding women, *Appl Nurs Res* 9(2):67–70, 1996.

Neelon VJ et al.: The Neecham confusion scale: construction, validation, and clinical testing, *Nurs Res* 45(6):324–330, 1996.

Oldham J, Howe T: The effectiveness of placebo muscle stimulation quadriceps muscle rehabilitation: a preliminary evaluation, *Clin Effectiv Nurs* 1:25–30, 1997.

Oppewal SR: Sister Elizabeth Kenney, an Australian nurse, and treatment of poliomyelitis victims, *Image: J Nurs Schol* 29:83–88, 1997.

Pell J: Cardiac rehabilitation: a review of its effectiveness, *Cor Health Care* 1:8–17, 1997.

Peterson FY, Kirchhoff KT: Analysis of the research about heparinized versus nonheparinized intravascular lines, *Heart Lung* 20:631–642, 1991.

Powell KB: Correlates of violent and nonviolent behavior among vulnerable inner-city youths, *Family Comm Health* 20(2):38–47, 1997.

Reese SM, Harkless G: Clinical methods: divergent themes in maternal experience in women older than 35 years, *Appl Nurs Res* 9(3):148–153, 1996.

Riordan J, Washburn J: Comparison of baccalaureate student lifestyle behaviors entering and completing the nursing program, *J Nurs Educ* 36:262–265, 1997.

Roberts KT, Whall A: Serenity as a goal for nursing practice, *Image: J Nurs Schol* 28(4):359–364, 1996.

Royal College of Nursing, Australia: Nursing Research: position statement, 1998, Canberra, Royal College of Nursing, Australia.

Russell KM, Champion VL: Health beliefs and social influence in home safety practice of mothers with preschool children, *Image: J Nurs Schol* 28(1):59–64, 1996.

Scannel-Desch EA: The lived experience of women military nurses in Vietnam during the Vietnam war, *Image: J Nurs Schol* 28(2):119–124, 1996.

Sherman DW: Nurses' willingness to care for AIDS patients and spirituality, social support, and death anxiety, *Image: J Nurs Schol* 28:205–213, 1996.



Shoaf J, Oliver S: Efficacy of normal saline injection with and without heparin for maintaining intermittent intravenous site, *Appl Nurs Res* 5(1):9–12, 1992.

Teel C et al.: Perspectives unifying symptom interpretation, *Image: J Nurs Schol* 29:175–181, 1997.

Waldenström U, Nilsson CA: No effect of birth centre care on either duration or experience of breast feeding, but more complications: findings from a randomised controlled trial, *Midwifery* 10:8–17, 1994.

Wellard S, Palaster L: An evaluation of two methods of pre-cannulation skin disinfection, *Aust J Adv Nurs* 14(1):3–7, 1996.

White GE, Thomson AN: As every good mother should: childhood immunisation in New Zealand: a qualitative study, *Health & Social Care* 3:73–82, 1995.

Wineman NM et al.: Relationships among illness uncertainty, stress, coping, and emotional well-being at entry into a clinical drug trial, *Appl Nurs Res* 9(2):53–60, 1996.

Zalon M: Pain in frail, elderly women after surgery, *Image: J Nurs Schol* 29:21–26, 1997.

Zerwic JJ, King KG, Wlasowsicz GS: Perceptions of patients with cardiovascular disease about the causes of coronary artery disease, *Heart Lung* 26:92–98, 1997.

# Appendix

## Chapter 1

### ACTIVITY ONE

**c  b  d  a  f  e**

### ACTIVITY TWO

Answers to the following questions may come from individuals, or following discussion in pairs, groups or formal class. There are no right or wrong answers. Answers will vary according to the discussion or group processes. The following are examples of answers, but are not exhaustive.

**a** Clinical nurse, community nurse, educator, manager, researcher, academic – and the various activities associated with these roles, including clinician, advocate, consultant, change agent.

**b** Answers will vary.

**c** Answers will vary. The important issue is the discussion, and a balance of positive and negative comments.

**d** Improve patient outcomes/nursing practice; highlight the uniqueness of nursing; validate change; support evidence-based practice; professional development; improve knowledge base of nurses and nursing.

**e** By disseminating research findings; providing access to knowledge (journals; Internet) for clinical nurses; improving research utilisation skills of nurses; support for improving practice according to the current knowledge base.

### ACTIVITY THREE

Answers will vary.

### ACTIVITY FOUR

**a** Aims and scope of the journals (taken from information stated in journal issues and/or websites).

*Contemporary Nurse*: Range of issues influencing professional nursing in Australia. Includes original research and reviews; current issues; quality undergraduate papers which contribute to nursing knowledge; descriptions of nursing practice.

*International Journal of Nursing Practice*: Original scholarly work that advances international understanding and development of nursing both as a profession and as an academic discipline. Includes research papers and professional discussion papers.

*Nursing Inquiry*: Contributions on philosophical, historical, methodological, ethical, policy and substantive issues relating to the everyday practice of nursing.

**b** Examples of other Australasian-based professional nursing journals (that is, no industrial/union orientation):

*Australian Critical Care*
*Australian Journal of Advanced Nursing*
*Australian Journal of Emergency Nursing*
*Australian Journal of Rural Health*
*Australian and New Zealand Journal of Mental Health Nursing*
*Collegian*.

# Chapter 2

## ACTIVITY ONE

**a** No. This was a descriptive, exploratory study, with objectives stated, not hypotheses (see page 565 of the textbook).

**b** No. No randomisation or interventions were conducted.

**c** No. Although not stated, the study surveyed MI patients regarding pre-hospital delay time and the factors impacting on the delay.

**d** No. Although the term convenience could be used appropriately to describe the sample.

**e** Yes. The Response to Symptoms Questionnaire was used (see page 567 of the textbook).



**f** No. Although validity of the above instrument is implied (see page 567 of the textbook).

**g** Yes. t-test/ANOVA, $\chi^2$, regression modelling (see page 567 of the textbook).

**h** Summary: This study would be categorised as quantitative, even though it meets only two of the seven criteria listed on page 40 of the textbook. It is not experimental or quasi-experimental (two of the specific types of quantitative research that are usually the only designs that include the terms hypotheses, control and treatment groups). The use of a questionnaire, numerical coding of the information and quantitative data analysis preclude a qualitative design. This study is a quantitative descriptive design (see page 183 of the textbook).

## ACTIVITY TWO

Go to the reference list for the Kermode article and check the source for Colaizzi, which is a chapter in an edited book by Valle and King. Check the library for the book, and/or use Colaizzi as a keyword for a search of CINAHL or PsycLIT (see page 106 of the textbook).

It is common to search for primary or secondary sources from the reference list to assist you in critically analysing the article of interest.

## ACTIVITY THREE

**a** Concepts: Coping style; quality of life; participation.

**b** Clarification of concepts: Ductal carcinoma in situ.

**c** Appropriateness of the assumptions or rationale: Focus on women with a specific diagnosis and exploration of similarities and differences in experiences were appropriate reasons for conducting the study using that design and method.

# Chapter 3

## ACTIVITY ONE

| | | | | |
|---|---|---|---|---|
| **a** | Yes; | Yes; | Yes; | Yes. |
| **b** | Yes; | Yes; | Yes; | Yes. |
| **c** | Yes; | No; | Yes; | Yes. |
| **d** | Yes; | Yes; | Yes; | Yes. |
| **e** | Yes; | Yes; | Yes; | Yes. |
| **f** | No; | No; | Yes; | Yes. |
| **g** | Yes; | No; | Yes; | Yes. |

## ACTIVITY TWO

**a** Independent variable: CRTs; dependent variable: birth defects.

**b** Independent variable: birth defects; dependent variable: independence–dependence conflicts.

**c** Independent variable: white wine; dependent variable: serum cholesterol level.

**d** Independent variable: type of recording (documentation); dependent variable: patient care.

**e** Independent variable: health profession (nursing; medicine); dependent variable: extended-role concept of nurses.

**f** Independent variable: sex, age, height, and weight; dependent variable: FEV1, haemoglobin concentration, food intake, serum glucose concentration, total serum cholesterol.

## ACTIVITY THREE

| | | |
|---|---|---|
| **a** Hr, DH | **b** Hr, DH | **c** RQ |
| **d** Hr, DH | **e** Hr, NDH | **f** RQ |

## ACTIVITY FOUR

**a** RQ Does the use of cathode ray terminals (CRTs) influence the incidence of birth defects?

Ho The use of CRTs by pregnant women has no effect on the incidence of birth defects.

**b** DH Individuals with birth defects have a higher incidence of independence–dependence conflicts than individuals without birth defects (as stated).

NDH There is a difference in the number of independence–dependence conflicts between individuals with and without birth defects.

Hr As stated.

RQ Do individuals with birth defects have a higher incidence of independence–dependence conflicts than those without birth defects?

Ho There is no difference in incidence of independence–dependence conflicts between individuals with and without birth defects.

**c** DH There is a positive relationship between daily moderate consumption of white wine and serum cholesterol levels.

NDH Daily moderate consumption of white wine influences serum cholesterol levels.

Hr There is a relationship between daily moderate consumption of white wine and serum cholesterol levels.

RQ As stated.

Ho There is no relationship between daily moderate consumption of white wine and serum cholesterol levels.

## ACTIVITY FIVE

Hypothesis 1:

- **a** Yes
- **b** Yes; IV– SPID; DV– dressing independence
- **c** Yes
- **d** Yes
- **e** Yes
- **f** Yes
- **g** Yes.

Hypothesis 2:

- **a** Yes
- **b** Yes
- **c** Yes
- **d** Yes
- **e** Yes
- **f** Yes
- **g** Yes.



## ACTIVITY SIX

The problem statement poses the question the researcher is asking. The hypothesis attempts to answer the question posed by the research problem. The problem does not predict a relationship between two or more variables.

# Chapter 4

## ACTIVITY ONE

A review of the literature contributes to the development of a strong knowledge base which is necessary for the conduct of research, the process of education and the practice of nursing. A critical review of the literature can:

- uncover new knowledge that can lead to the development, validation or refinement of theories

- uncover knowledge about particular topics, concepts or problems
- reveal appropriate research questions for the discipline of nursing
- provide the latest knowledge for education purposes
- provide research findings that can lead to changes in clinical practice, especially for the development of research-based interventions/practice protocols.

## ACTIVITY TWO

- Determines what is known and not known about a subject, concept or problem.
- Determines gaps, consistencies and inconsistencies in the literature about a subject, concept or problem.
- Discovers unanswered questions about a subject, concept or problem.
- Discovers conceptual traditions used to examine problems.
- Uncovers new practice intervention(s) or gains support for current intervention(s).
- Promotes development of new or revised practice protocols, policies and projects/activities related to nursing practice and the discipline.

## ACTIVITY THREE

**a** D **b** C **c** D **d** D **e** C **f** D

## ACTIVITY FOUR

There is a great range of scholarly nursing journals available, including the following, that could be used to answer the question:

*Advances in Nursing Science; AORN Journal; Applied Nursing Research; Australian Critical Care; Australian Journal of Advanced Nursing; Computers in Nursing; Heart & Lung; Holistic Nursing Practice; Image: Journal of Nursing Scholarship; Clinical Nursing Research; Nursing Inquiry; Journal of Nursing Education; Journal of Professional Nursing; Nurse Educator; Nursing Research; Nursing Science Quarterly; Research in Nursing and Health; Western Journal of Nursing Research.*

## ACTIVITY FIVE

**a** ***Barclay et al.(1996)***

No section heading is given. The authors refer to the context of men's experiences as expectant fathers but do not extensively explore the literature related to the context. This is a typical introduction to a qualitative study using grounded theory methodology. In this type of research the author will bring some knowledge of the literature to the study but does not usually do an exhaustive search. Instead the researcher allows theory to emerge from the data, a process that is described in detail in Chapter 9 in the textbook.

***Dracup et al. (1997)***

No section heading is given, however the opening paragraphs clearly provide an overview of the problem and what is known and not known about it. The pathophysiological (theoretical) underpinnings of the importance of reducing delay is identified. The review summarises the outcomes of earlier studies on factors related to prehospital delay, but it does not refer to the design or methods of previous studies.

**b** ***Barclay et al. (1996)***

Yes. The authors point out that despite research into the needs of expectant fathers, the health care system continues to focus on women's needs. It neglects the dyadic context in which most women give birth which has the effect of limiting the effectiveness of antenatal preparation for parenting.

***Dracup et al. (1997)***

Yes. The authors explain that while previous studies have revealed the factors contributing to delay, it is not known if these factors/characteristics are similar in the Australian population. They point out the importance of this information for the design of appropriate education programs.

**c** ***Dracup et al. (1997)***

Yes.

**d** ***Dracup et al. (1997)***

With the exception of two dated 1977 and 1978, the remaining references range from 1986 to 1995, although the Simoons et al. reference is not dated. The earlier references refer to seminal work that supports assertions made by the authors in the text. The references do portray the development of research over time, beginning with work related to the effectiveness of early thrombolytic therapy in the treatment of myocardial infarction. They go on to studies related to the concept of delay in seeking treatment and the reasons/factors/behaviours that are associated with delay. This is followed by work that explores change in perceptions and behaviours. However, while the flow of the research story is evident, the dates of the references do not follow chronologically. There are no references to qualitative studies.



## ACTIVITY SIX

**a** S P S S P P P

**b** False

**c** 1982

**d** CINAHL. MEDLINE does not contain all the nursing references that CINAHL does.

**e**
- www.scu.edu.au/schools/nhcp/aejne/aejnehpa.htm
- www.joannabriggs.edu.au and the 'What's New?' section of the Home Page
- nursing sites on the World Wide Web

**f** Riley JM, Mahoney MA, Fry ST, Field L.

**g** Bedsores; pressure ulcers; pressure sores; decubitus ulcers.

## ACTIVITY SEVEN

**a** D; P **b** C; P **c** D; P **d** D; S **e** D; P

## ACTIVITY EIGHT

**a** What is the source of the material? Look at the last term in the URL address for US sources and the second last when the source is outside the US, to find the organisational name (it is three letters long). Possibilities include: *com* for commercial organisation, *edu* for educational institution, *gov* for government body, *int* for international organisation, *net* for networking organisation, and *org* for anything else.

You can feel comfortable with information gathered from an edu or gov source such as www.joannabriggs.edu.au that takes you to the Joanna Briggs Institute for Evidence Based Nursing and Midwifery in Adelaide, or from www.anci.org.au which will take you to The Australian Nursing Council Inc., or http://cinahl.com for CINAHL information systems based in the US.

**b** Is the source a well-respected medical or nursing institution or government agency, or is the source an individual putting out his/her own opinion? Critique the source.

**c** Is the name of the researcher, or researchers, and their qualifications given?

**d** Is there a mechanism given to obtain further information about the study or the information presented?

**e** Is enough data given in the WWW publication to make a critical analysis in the same way as an analysis can be made about a research article using the critiquing criteria in the textbook? Note: In a refereed, professional journal there are usually two or three independent nursing experts in the field who have reviewed the article in a blind review process to determine that the material merits publication.

# Chapter 5



## ACTIVITY ONE

Inductive thinking: Moves from the specific to the general (conclusions are developed from specific observations).

Deductive thinking: Moves from the general to the specific (predictions are developed from known relationships).

## ACTIVITY TWO

**a** Learned helplessness, self-esteem, depression, health practices, homeless women (Flynn, 1997).

**b** Illness, uncertainty, stress, coping, emotional well-being, clinical drug trial (Wineman et al., 1996).

**c** Social support, intervention, pregnancy outcome, lower income, African-American women (Bolla et al., 1996).

**d** Violent behaviour, non-violent behaviour, vulnerable, inner-city youths (Powell, 1997).

**e** Verbal abuse, staff nurses, physicians, stress coping. Prevalence and consequences could also be listed as concepts especially if you think of them as capturing an idea (Manderino et al., 1997).

## ACTIVITY THREE

**a** Answers will vary

**b** • There are no 'correct' answers for this question. Rather, the thinking that you do to reach a consensus definition is the 'correct answer'.

- Answers will vary. An argument could be made for the following to be considered constructs: illness uncertainty; social support intervention; verbal abuse.

## ACTIVITY FOUR

Barclay et al. (1996): As a grounded theory study, no pre-determined concepts of interest were defined.

Waldenstöm and Nilsson (1994): Birth centre care. Encouragement of natural childbirth and emphasis ... on continuity of care, parental involvement and support in labour (see page 540 of the textbook).

Kermode (1995): AIDS-defining illness. The first opportunistic infection or condition experienced by an HIV-positive person ... (see page 553 of the textbook).

Dracup et al. (1997): MI – chest pain, ECG changes, serum enzyme changes (see page 566 of the textbook); delay in treatment – cognitive, symptom appraisal and social factors (see page 567 of the textbook).

## ACTIVITY FIVE

**a** Operational definition
**b** Concept
**c** Conceptual definition
**d** Operational definition
**e** Concept or construct
**f** Construct
**g** Conceptual definition
**h** Variable
**i** Hypothesis



## ACTIVITY SIX

**a** Birth centre care; breast feeding.

**b** Example answers:

*Breast feeding*

- Many maternal factors are associated with duration of breast feeding – age, education, social class, attitudes.
- Information about breast feeding, childbirth education and support also influence practices.
- Hospital factors may also influence breast feeding, for example, suckling practices, rooming-in, length of hospital stay.

*Delivery care*

- The aims of birth centre care are continuity of care, parental involvement and women self-care.
- Standard care involves antenatal classes, delivery and postpartum care with input from different sets of midwives.
- Differences in practices between the two types of care were evident.

**c** Deductive.

**d** Yes, 'birth centre care was more beneficial for the outcome of breast feeding than standard maternity care'.

**e** None of the above.

**f** Location and process of delivery in relation to impact on duration and experience of breast feeding.

# Chapter 6

## ACTIVITY ONE

- **a** The end result of the research endeavour must not be at the expense of compromising the tenets of informed consent and patients' rights. Researchers and caregivers of research subjects, such as patients, must be fully committed to taking every precaution to protect people being studied from physical or mental harm or discomfort. In this context the ends do not justify the means.
- **b** The National Health and Medical Research Council (NHMRC).
- **c** The principles laid down by the Nuremburg Code and the Declaration of Helsinki.
- **d** http://www.health.gov.au/nhmrc/ethics/humanexp/contents.htm or from any Institutional Ethics Committee.
- **e** Institutional Ethics Committees review all research projects to ensure that they adhere to current ethical guidelines and that standards are met in regard to the protection of the rights of human subjects. They monitor ongoing projects to ensure that the guidelines for ethical conduct are followed and they maintain records of research conducted at the particular institution.
- **f** The areas of biotechnology (for example, genetic engineering); the use of animals for research; foetal tissue research; and the use of women who are of childbearing potential as subjects in drug/therapeutic studies.
- **g** The right to self-determination; the right to privacy and dignity; the right to anonymity or confidentiality; the right to fair treatment; and the right to protection from discomfort and harm.



## ACTIVITY TWO

Respect for persons; beneficence; justice.

## ACTIVITY THREE

### *Barclay et al. (1996)*

The authors mention that the study was explained by the researchers and information sheets were distributed the week before data collection. They describe the opportunity given to couples to attend 'their conventional classes instead of a focus group but all the men consented to their inclusion in the study'. There is no mention of whether the consent was in writing. Also there is no mention of women attending the 'conventional classes' on their own, or where and when the men received their antenatal information.

The study was approved by the Area Health Service Institutional Ethics Committee and the authors maintain that the 'participants' anonymity was strictly observed'.

### *Waldenström and Nilsson (1994)*

The authors mention that a 'willingness to participate in the research project with random allocation' was a prerequisite for joining the trial. How the 'willingness' was established is not evident. There is no indication that informed consent or ethics approval had been obtained. This may be a stylistic consideration of the journal, an editorial decision of the authors, a matter of space constraints, or simply forgotten or neglected.

***Kermode (1995)***

Under the heading of 'The Participants', the author mentions that 'participants signed a consent form after being informed about the nature of the study and assured of confidentiality'. It is unclear whether the information was verbal or in written form. Approval to conduct the study was given by the 'hospital's research and ethics committee'.

***Dracup et al. (1997)***

Under the heading of 'Methods', the authors indicate that participants in the study 'gave written informed consent' and that the project had been reviewed and approved by 'the study hospitals' as well as the University of Technology, Sydney. (Depending on the particular University, when research projects are undertaken by academics and/or research students in the clinical setting, it is necessary to obtain approval from the Institutional Ethics Committee of the relevant University as well as the clinical facility/Area Health Service).

## ACTIVITY FOUR

The elderly, indigenous populations, children, pregnant women, the unborn, those who are emotionally or physically disabled, prisoners, the deceased, students and people with AIDS.

## ACTIVITY FIVE



**a** The subjects in this study are students. They are a vulnerable population and, therefore, extra precautions must be undertaken to protect their rights.

**b** The subjects in this study are adolescents, who make up a vulnerable population, and prisoners, who are both a captive and convenient population, thus extra precautions would need to be taken to protect their rights.

## ACTIVITY SIX

**a** Core committee membership: one layman; one laywoman; one minister of religion; one lawyer; one medical graduate with research experience. The NHMRC are currently reviewing their core membership and are considering the inclusion of a nurse as a core member.

**b** Note: Each student's answer may vary. For example, at the University of Sydney the composition of the Institutional Ethics Committee is as follows: two laymen; one laywoman; one minister of religion; two lawyers; one nurse; one physiotherapist; one anaesthetist; one epidemiologist; one psychologist; a doctor experienced in qualitative research; a manager (of Ethics and Biosafety Administration); and a secretary. Additional members are seconded as appropriate for clinical trials.

For the Central Sydney Area Health Service (Royal Prince Alfred Hospital zone) the composition of the Institutional Ethics Committee includes: two laymen; two laywomen; one minister of religion; one lawyer; one psychologist; one nurse; one physiologist; one general surgeon; one pharmacist; one paediatrician; one respiratory physician; one immunologist; and a secretary/manager.

## ACTIVITY SEVEN

### *Consent form*

I understand that if I agree to participate I will be involved in a research project that is investigating patient's experiences of nursing interventions during hospitalisation with an AIDS-defining illness, which is being conducted by M. Kermode.

I understand that the purposes of the study are to explore patients' experiences of being diagnosed with AIDS and their perceptions of nursing interventions that are helpful and unhelpful during hospitalisation.

It is not expected that my involvement will take very long.

I understand that I will take part in an audiotaped interview with the researcher which will take place just before being discharged. I may be asked to participate in a follow-up interview.

My participation does not involve any foreseeable risks or discomfort and while I may not benefit directly from the research, others may in the future.

My participation is voluntary and I may choose to not participate or to withdraw at any time without jeopardising my future treatment.

I understand that my identity will not be revealed and that no identifiable aspects of my interview will be made public.

If I have any queries about the research I can contact M. Kermode on number _____. In the event of any concerns that I might have about the overall conduct of the research I understand that I can contact the Institutional Ethics Committee secretary on number _____ .

I will receive a copy of this consent form.

Date ________________ Patient __________________

Witness _______________ Investigator ______________



## ACTIVITY EIGHT

- **a** One ethical principle guiding research is beneficence. This imparts an obligation to do no harm and maximise possible benefits. Therefore, it would not be ethical to conduct an experimental study at this time. Instead, perhaps conduct a descriptive or qualitative study describing the patients and their symptoms and the treatments being used, and then begin to identify all the variables involved.
- **b** The population of interest is children, who are one of the vulnerable groups, so extra precautions must be taken to protect their rights. However, at that time (1942), guidelines had not yet been developed that identified children as a vulnerable population nor had the Nuremburg Code, which was the original code of ethics for research that was developed after the Second World War. In research involving children, parental consent is required.
- **c** The study would have to be descriptive, or qualitative, describing in detail all the variables involved.

# Chapter 7

## ACTIVITY ONE

- **a** Design
- **b** Accuracy
- **c** Control
- **d** Feasibility
- **e** Homogeneity
- **f** Random sampling
- **g** Internal validity
- **h** External validity

## ACTIVITY TWO

- **a** Maturation. The mothers' confidence could be increased by any number of factors, including the act of caring for the baby during the month. The time of measurement could be at discharge. Use of a control group would strengthen the study.
- **b** Instrumentation. The use of standardised calibrated equipment and training for the volunteers would increase the internal validity of the study.
- **c** History. The increase in taxes could account for a decrease in the rate of cigarette smoking. Use of a control group and randomisation would improve the interpretation of the findings.
- **d** Selection bias. The differences in smoking cessation rates could be attributed to a number of motivational factors. Random assignment to smoking cessation groups is needed to strengthen the design.
- **e** Mortality. The program is not successful for young unemployed women with children. It is important to consider the characteristics of the final study sample when interpreting the results.
- **f** Testing. Taking the test repeatedly may be the factor leading to an increase in confidence and accuracy, rather than the teaching program. The use of different measuring instruments (exams) may be necessary.



## ACTIVITY THREE

- **a** Hospital obstetric care and an in-hospital birth centre in Stockholm.
- **b** Low-risk pregnant women living in the Greater Stockholm area who were Swedish-speaking and willing to participate in either mode of care.
- **c** Random allocation to birth centre care (treatment group) or standard obstetric care (control group).
- **d** None. Information was provided on the sampling methods and sample selection.
- **e** Yes, there was homogeneity between the two groups for the characteristics age, length of gestation, parity, civil status, ethnic background, education and attitudes to breast feeding.
- **f** Variables were measured by self-report questionnaire. The exact items were not stated in the paper, but were related to the rates, duration, women's experiences, complications, and satisfaction with breast feeding.

**g** Standard obstetric care.

## ACTIVITY FOUR

**a** Yes, a randomised controlled trial is the 'gold standard' for comparing the outcomes of two different interventions.

**b** The researchers used control methods appropriate for experimental research, including random assignment, a control group of usual care, and an experimental group to test the hypotheses.

**c** The study was feasible by using a convenience sample of women booked for delivery.

**d** There is logical flow of the design between various sections of the study. Factors influencing breast feeding were identified, as well as the gap in knowledge regarding whether the place of birth has any impact on breast-feeding behaviour. The null hypotheses were that there were no differences between birth centre care and standard obstetric care for the rates, duration, women's experiences or complications of breast-feeding.

**e** Threats to internal validity include any extraneous variables that could influence the results of the study, such as selection bias, mortality, maturation, instrumentation, testing and history.

**f** Internal validity was maintained through control such as inviting participation from women interested in birth centre care (minimising selection bias – see page 187 of the textbook). However, there was evidence of greater than 50 per cent study drop-out (mortality) from the first to the third measurement. There was also a potential threat regarding instrumentation – the questionnaire was not fully described and no pilot test appeared to be conducted.

**g** Threats to external validity could include effects of selection, testing or reactivity.

**h** External validity was maintained through randomisation and a control group, a sufficient sample size to detect clinical differences in breast-feeding rates, and a protocol to avoid effects of testing and reactivity. The results are generalisable to other similar patient populations.



## ACTIVITY FIVE

**a** To identify factors which contribute to the delay in seeking treatment for patients with acute myocardial infarction (AMI).

**b** Two teaching hospitals and one district hospital in Sydney.

**c** 317 patients with a confirmed diagnosis of AMI.

**d** Sample criteria were: able to read and write English, lived independently, were alert and oriented, were within twenty-four to seventy-two hours of admission with a diagnosis of AMI.

**e** A 'response to symptoms' questionnaire with six domains was modified to focus on decisions to seek care for AMI symptoms. The questionnaire was administered by an interview in hospital. Patient medical records were also reviewed for additional data.

# Chapter 8

## ACTIVITY ONE

- **a** Solomon four-group design
- **b** Time series design
- **c** After-only experiment
- **d** After-only non-equivalent control group design
- **e** True experiment
- **f** Non-equivalent control group design

## ACTIVITY TWO

**a** Randomisation: Subjects were randomly assigned to one of two groups. The women selected an envelope out of a group of approximately fifty in the birth centre which allocated them to birth centre care or standard obstetric care.
Control: Standard obstetric care served as the control group.
Manipulation: The independent (explanatory) variable was the type and setting of peri-natal care; birth centre care was the experimental group.

**b** The study found that there were no differences in breast-feeding rates or duration, although complications were increased in the birth centre group.

**c** Another factor could account for the differences.



**d** It would have been a descriptive study.

## ACTIVITY THREE

**a**

| | PRETEST | TEACHING | POST-TEST |
|---|---|---|---|
| Group A | X | X | X |
| Group B | | X | X |
| Group C | X | | X |
| Group D | | | X |

Note: Groups may be arranged in any order, but the four group pattern must be followed.

**b** Nurses would be randomly assigned to each of the groups by using a table of random numbers or computer random assignment.

**c** The Pain Knowledge and Attitudes Questionnaire would be used as a pretest.

**d** The teaching program is the experimental treatment.

**e** The Pain Knowledge and Attitudes Questionnaire is the post-test (outcome measure).

**f** The Solomon four-group design is ideal for experimental studies in which the pretest might affect the outcome. In this case, the questionnaire might change nurses' knowledge and attitudes about pain management. The researcher will be able to compare results for nurses receiving the teaching and not receiving the teaching with and without the pretest.

**g** This type of design is particularly effective in ruling out threats to internal validity that the before and after groups may experience. It is effective for highly sensitive issues that might be affected by simply completing a questionnaire as a baseline pretest.

**h** A disadvantage of the Solomon four-group design is that a large number of subjects must be available for assignment into the four groups.

## ACTIVITY FOUR

**a**
- After-only non-equivalent control group.
- Subjects were available for the study; study was practical and feasible.
- Lack of ability to establish a cause and effect relationship; lack of generalisability to a larger population because of no randomisation.

**b**
- True experiment.
- Cause and effect relationship is clearer, as other factors that could affect results are controlled for through random assignment to treatment and control groups.
- Cost and complexity of strict control measures and the large sample size necessary.

**c**
- Quasi-experimental, non-equivalent control group.
- Not possible to randomly assign subjects to groups, but use of a pretest and post-test was possible.
- Many factors could affect performance. It is therefore difficult to conclude that the accelerated students have higher performance in other situations. Sample size of groups were small for comparative purposes. Groups were similar demographically, although traditional students worked more hours and studied less – this may have affected their results.

**d**
- Time series.
- Not possible to use random assignment in this study, but use of a group with similar characteristics except for irritability, allowed for comparisons. In longitudinal studies, each subject can be compared with themselves over time to observe trends.
- Cause and effect relationships are more difficult to determine when random assignment is not conducted. Careful examination of the comparison between groups is necessary to determine if other factors affect the differences observed.

## ACTIVITY FIVE

**a** Experimental: Random assignment; control group; intervention to one group.
**b** Quasi-experimental: No random assignment.
**c** Experimental: Random assignment; control group; intervention to one group.
**d** Experimental: Random assignment; control group; intervention to one group.

## ACTIVITY SIX

**a** Survey
**b** Longitudinal
**c** Correlational
**d** Ex post facto
**e** Cross-sectional
**f** Correlational
**g** Longitudinal
**h** Survey
**i** Cross-sectional
**j** Cross-sectional

## ACTIVITY SEVEN

| | | ADVANTAGE(S) | DISADVANTAGE(S) |
|---|---|---|---|
| **a** | Correlation studies | A3 | D1, D3, D4, D7 |
| **b** | Cross-sectional | A1 | D2, D5 |
| **c** | Descriptive/exploratory | A1 | D1, D5 |
| **d** | Ex post facto | A4 | D1, D2, D3, D4, D5, D7 |
| **e** | Longitudinal | A2, A6 | D2, D8 |
| **f** | Prediction studies | A5 | D1 |
| **g** | Prospective | A2, A7 | D3, D4, D7, D8 |
| **h** | Retrospective | A4 | D1, D2, D3, D4, D5, D7 |
| **i** | Survey | A1 | D5, D7 |

## ACTIVITY EIGHT

**a** M
**b** C, D
**c** S, C
**d** MA
**e** L, S
**f** D, R
**g** S, C

# Chapter 9



## ACTIVITY ONE

**a** Quantitative
**b** Qualitative
**c** Qualitative
**d** Quantitative
**e** Qualitative
**f** Quantitative
**g** Quantitative
**h** Qualitative
**i** Qualitative

## ACTIVITY TWO

**a** Data saturation
**b** Theoretical sampling
**c** Etic view
**d** Bracketed
**e** Emic view
**f** Domains
**g** Key informants
**h** Case study method
**i** Secondary sources
**j** Grounded theory method

## ACTIVITY THREE

***Identifying the phenomenon***

Phenomenology: Study of day-to-day existence for a particular group of individuals.
Grounded theory: Interested in social processes from the perspective of human interactions.
Ethnography: Study of the complex cultural aspects related to a phenomenon.
Historical: An approach for understanding a past event.

### *Structuring the study*

The research question:

- queries the lived experience
- includes questions which address basic social processes and tend to be action oriented
- includes questions about lifeways or patterns of behaviour within a social context
- includes questions which are implicit and embedded in the phenomenon studied.

The researcher:

- has a bracketed perspective (however this notion is currently being challenged)
- brings some knowledge of the literature although an exhaustive review is not done
- attempts to make sense of the world from the insider's point of view
- has an understanding of the information without imposing an interpretation.

Sample:

- is living or has lived the experience
- is experiencing the circumstance/events/incidents related to the social process
- is the cultural group living the phenomenon
- is the historical data source(s).

**b** ***Barclay et al. (1996)***

By referring to the social processes associated with male identity and relationships in the context of pregnancy the problem of men's experiences is highlighted.

***Kermode (1995)***

Referring to the patient's perspective as an important source of information, the author explored their subjective, or lived, experience of being diagnosed with AIDS, and their experiences of nursing interventions during hospitalisation.



## ACTIVITY FOUR

**a** The impact of pregnancy and parenting on the male partner.

**b** When critical thinking is involved, then it is possible that several different ideas may emerge as ways this information might be used. For example, the review could increase nurses'/midwives' understanding of how men can be affected when their partner becomes pregnant and help them to appreciate that they have important needs. Given the greater involvement of men in parenting in recent times, it is necessary that their needs and concerns are addressed to a similar extent as those of women.

**c** The authors use the literature at the beginning of the article to 'set the scene' by highlighting the impact of pregnancy and parenting on the male partner. In the discussion section the authors use literature from previous work to add meaning to some of the categories that emerged as well as to substantiate or support the findings. Being able to locate some of the findings in the wider literature base helps to contextualise the information and to confirm, or help to establish, the knowledge base. The process of locating findings in the wider literature base in the discussion section is not unique to the qualitative method. The difference is that an extensive review of the literature is not undertaken at the outset of a grounded theory study, but rather when the data have revealed themes and categories which are then explored through the literature.

## ACTIVITY FIVE

| | | |
|---|---|---|
| **a** D | **b** C | **c** B |
| **d** A | **e** A | **f** B |
| **g** C | **h** D | **i** D |
| **j** A | **k** C | **l** C |
| **m** D | **n** C | **o** B |
| **p** A | **q** A (could also be true of B or C) | **r** A (could also be true of B, C or D) |
| **s** C | **t** D (could also be true of A or C) | **u** C (could also be true of A) |
| **v** B | **w** C | |

## ACTIVITY SIX

**a** Phenomenological
**b** Nursing practice
**c** Convenience sampling

## ACTIVITY SEVEN

The items in this question could have a variety of answers depending on which method was chosen.



# Chapter 10

## ACTIVITY ONE

| | | |
|---|---|---|
| **a** P | **b** N | **c** P |
| **d** N | **e** N | **f** P |
| **g** P | | |

## ACTIVITY TWO

**a** Quota sampling
**b** Systematic sampling
**c** Simple random sampling
**d** Convenience sampling
**e** Cluster sampling
**f** Purposive sampling
**g** Stratified random sampling

## ACTIVITY THREE

**a** Yes. Inclusion criteria were stated (see page 542 of the textbook).
**b** Partially. No high-risk pregnant women were included.
**c** Non-purposive sample. Convenience.
**d** Yes. Sample sizes were calculated according to a stated clinical difference between groups (see page 542 of the textbook).

## ACTIVITY FOUR

| | | |
|---|---|---|
| **a** True | **b** True | **c** False |
| **d** False | **e** True | **f** True |

## ACTIVITY FIVE

**1** The researchers described the sample in terms of age, gender, marital status, education status and socio-economic status. Further clinical variables were described (previous chest pain, hypertension, diabetes mellitus). Delay time prehospital was a major variable under examination in this study.

**2** The description of the sample allows some inferences to be made about the population parameters. The subjects were predominantly older married males with a diversity of educational and socio-economic backgrounds (see page 568 of the textbook).

**3** The sample represents patients admitted with a diagnosis of Acute Myocardial Infarction (AMI) who are English-speaking and have no complicating illnesses. Hence, there may be limitations in representativeness related to individuals who were non-English speaking, not cognitively responsive within the seventy-two hours, and/or had the presence of multiple diseases. In addition, the study precluded individuals who did not survive to hospital admission. Some information on the number of patients with AMI who were excluded from all causes would have been useful in determining the representativeness of the sample.

**4** Eligibility criteria included the ability to read and write English, living independently, no cancer or complicating illnesses, alert and oriented, and were within twenty-four to seventy-two hours of admission with a diagnosis of AMI.



**5** Delimitations were included in the inclusion criteria, specifically for the diagnosis of AMI: duration of chest pain longer than twenty minutes; serial electrocardiograph (ECG) evidence of Q waves in at least two leads; elevated serum enzymes (CK-MB). Patients with Non-Q wave MIs and those mechanically ventilated were excluded.

**6** It would be possible to replicate the study population, as the sample was described in some detail.

**7** The convenience sample was drawn from patients admitted to three hospitals during a six month period. This sampling method was appropriate because it sampled from the catchment area of a particular health service, and 'self-selection' was not an issue in this case (see page 268 of the textbook).

**8** There may be some bias if there were some unique characteristics for this geographical area. In addition, the issue of no non-English speaking subjects has been previously raised, and no information on the characteristics of the non-subject patients or the general AMI patients was given.

**9** There was no information given on sample size requirements, although this study was descriptive and correlational in design. A six month data collection period was apparent. The sample size of 317 patients appeared appropriate given that significant results were reported. There was no substantiation for the sample size given.

**10** The procedure included discussion of project approval by the Institutional Ethics

Committees (study hospitals and the University of Technology, Sydney), and written informed consent from the patients.

**11** The researchers reported that the inclusion criteria and resulting sample did not represent all patients with AMI. No methodological limitations were discussed.

**12** The researchers discussed the differences in definitions for time of delay, when compared to previous studies (see page 569 of the textbook). Replication of the study in different settings was not discussed in this paper.

# Chapter 11

## ACTIVITY ONE

### *Barclay et al. (1996)*

**a** An interview measure.

**b** Focus group interviews were appropriate in this context. It provided an opportunity for the members to participate in a conversation that was led by someone who had experienced the circumstances under investigation. The authors reported that the men were comfortable about disclosing information about their emotional and sexual relationships and were assisted by the group processes. It is possible that the participants were more likely to share their feelings in this context than if they were interviewed individually.



**c** Open-ended.

**d** Gender specific within-group homogeneity is important because it means that the group members are as comparable as possible in regard to the study topic. It was necessary in this context because the experience of sharing a first pregnancy in a relationship is potentially quite different to subsequent pregnancies. Only one of the group members had some previous experience, but this pregnancy was the first in the present relationship.

### *Waldenström and Nilsson (1994)*

**a** Questionnaire measure; records or available data.

**b** In this randomised control trial questionnaires are appropriate because of the size of the sample and the nature of the process, that is three episodes of data collection. Such a large volume of data is more manageable when it is able to be entered onto a spread-sheet and statistically analysed. The research design is strengthened when using this approach because the researcher aims to draw conclusions about cause and effect relationships.

The hospital records were an appropriate source of information related to obstetric medication and transfers of women in the experimental group.

**c** There were three episodes of data collection, using a questionnaire for each. The first, at the time of enrolment into the trial, collected information about demographics and attitudes towards breast feeding; the second was at two months after the birth; and the third was at twelve months after the birth. There were 617 women enrolled into the experimental group (EG) at the beginning and 613 into the control group (CG). At the third data collection there were less than 50 per cent of women in each of the original groups (EG – 299 and CG – 275). One of the problems of longitudinal studies is the mortality threat to internal validity. Such a large loss of subjects from the first data collection point to the third could affect the results of the study because it is not known if those remaining are similar to those who 'dropped out'. In addition, while the frequency of missing data was acknowledged as low, not all women responded to all the questions in the three questionnaires which, although minimal, has the potential to affect results.

Although the authors identify the major aspects of each questionnaire, their development as data collection instruments is not described and there is no indication of a pilot test. It is not known how many items were in each questionnaire or whether the respondents had any difficulty in understanding some of the items. Therefore the reliability and validity of the instruments is open to question.

**d** Attitudes to breast-feeding; belief in the importance of breast feeding (Table 1); experience of midwife during labour (Table 2); physical well-being; and anxiety (Figure 2).

### *Kermode (1995)*

**a** An interview measure.

**b** Semi-structured in-depth interviews are an appropriate method for collecting the kind of data required from the subjects in this study. However, another method is possible if the researcher remained with the primary aim of the study only – to explore patients' perceptions of nursing interventions that were helpful and unhelpful during hospitalisation. This information could have been collected using a questionnaire with a list of relevant nursing interventions and asking the respondent to identify whether they were helpful or not (a space would need to be included where respondents could add interventions that were not listed). But the data would not have been as rich and meaningful. The secondary aim of the study was to develop an understanding of the experience of being diagnosed with AIDS, and the interview method is entirely appropriate in this context.

**c** Follow-up interviews were conducted with five of the eight participants to ensure that the researcher's understanding and interpretation of the data was compatible with the participants. This process helps to eliminate bias and establish rigour in a qualitative study.

**d** Structured interviews are usually conducted using an ordered questionnaire with a fixed number of alternative responses and the respondent is asked to choose the response closest to the right one. The items should be grammatically correct, free of jargon and value laden terms, not open to alternative interpretations and in a language that is understandable to respondents. The interviewer should present the questions in the same way and the same order for each respondent.

Semi-structured interviews involve the use of several open-ended questions that are focused and specific. Participants are able to respond freely to the question and subsequent questions may arise. Prompts may be used to facilitate the direction of the interview. The researcher will usually bring the participant back to the issue if the dialogue moves from the topic.

An unstructured interview (or conversation) can be initiated by a broad question that allows the participant to talk freely about their experiences, feelings, attitudes and thoughts in relation to the topic. The researcher is led by the participant and subsequent questions relate directly to the dialogue.

### *Dracup et al. (1997)*

**a** An interview measure; a questionnaire measure; records or available data.

**b** The researchers used medical records to obtain socio-demographic and clinical data including information related to the time of onset of symptoms and arrival time at hospital. Data related to six domains involving the cognitive, emotional and social processes surrounding the decision to seek treatment were collected using the content of an established questionnaire. However, in order to gather additional information relative to the study the questionnaire was modified. The resulting instrument was appropriate to the purpose of the study. In order to compare the written record with the patient's account of symptoms and time of onset the 'patients were carefully interviewed', but it is not clear whether the information obtained was part of the questionnaire data or separate interview data. Notwithstanding this, the authors described the data collection process in appropriate detail.



**c** The nature of MI symptoms; time from onset of symptoms to arrival at hospital; factors contributing to the delay in seeking treatment following the onset; the response of others to symptoms; and the patient's response to symptoms.

**d** Respondents would be able to ask for clarification of any unclear items. This method of data collection represents a structured interview approach and the data collectors would need to ask the questions in the same way and in the same order for each respondent so that inter-rater reliability would not be threatened.

## ACTIVITY TWO

| | | |
|---|---|---|
| **a** Physiological | **b** Reactivity | **c** Interviews |
| **d** Records | **e** Questionnaire | **f** Objectivity, consistency |
| **g** Concealment | **h** Inter-rater reliability | **i** Operationalisation |
| **j** Likert scale | **k** Content analysis | **l** Pilot |

## ACTIVITY THREE

**a** This study could involve observing the influence of different testing skills on the behaviour of pre-schoolers being given a cognitive skill-based instrument. A one-way window could be used to collect the data.

**b** Consent from the parents and the institution/agency in which the testing would take place is necessary.

**c** Concealment with intervention.

## ACTIVITY FOUR

Physiological measures would be of minimal use since the data being sought would not involve actual measures of the residents' physiological status. There is no real interest in current blood pressure, temperature, urinary output, etc.

Observation is a possibility, for example sitting in an emergency room and observing the types of health care problems and concerns that people bring. You would need to think about whether or not this would be observation without concealment, and consider the notion of what is private information and what is public domain information.

It might be possible to use questionnaires to collect data from all types of health care providers. This could yield a lot of data in a short time. But you would need to consider how busy these people would be and what would be the probability of their filling out the questionnaire.

Perhaps an interview. Costly in terms of researcher time, but could provide the information in more detail because participants could be asked to expand upon specific items. But who would be appropriate to interview and the question of access arises.

Information from the people who actually live in the community is needed. How to reach a cross section of those individuals? Perhaps a telephone call, but what of those without a telephone?

It might be useful to consult the census data in order to obtain a clearer picture of what needs to be dealt with. Morbidity and mortality data will have been collected by the health department. Existing records could be used to firstly get a sense of what the parameters of 'health' are in the community. Then find out who knows the most about the area and arrange some interviews with these individuals. These would be semi-structured interviews with open-ended items to encourage the sharing of as much information as possible. A means of collecting data from a variety of health care users could be explored, for example surveys in the waiting-room of various health care agencies, perhaps some people at a shopping plaza, a market, or country show.

One data collection instrument would not be sufficient to collect all the information needed to address the purpose of the study.

## ACTIVITY FIVE

**a** The instrument has objectivity, sensitivity and precision.
**b** Operationalisation.
**c** All of the above.
**d** Consistency.
**e** Inter-rater reliability.
**f** Whenever expense is a concern for the researcher; when a researcher is interested in obtaining information directly from the subjects; when the researcher needs to collect data from a large group of subjects that are not easily accessible.
**g** All of the above.
**h** It contains open-ended items.
**i** All of the above.

# Chapter 12

## ACTIVITY ONE

**a** S. Avoided by correct calibration of the weight scale.

**b** S. Decrease error by providing instructions, ensuring confidentiality of responses, or other means which would allow students to answer openly and honestly.

**c** R. Decrease error by training the evaluators and using explicit protocols for assessing wound healing.

**d** R. Anxiety may alter the test responses. Attempt to decrease anxiety by explanation, addressing concerns or providing comfort measures.

## ACTIVITY TWO

**a** Content; criterion; construct.

**b** Rating from a panel of experts.

**c** Criterion or concurrent.

**d** Construct.

**e** Multi-trait–multi-method

**f** Face.

**g** Hypothesis testing; convergent and divergent; contrasted groups; factor analysis.

**h** Convergent



**i** Divergent.

## ACTIVITY THREE

**a** Stability; homogeneity; equivalence.

**b** Test–retest methods would involve giving the same test again at a later date and seeing if the scores from the two tests were highly correlated. Parallel or alternate forms, such as alternate versions of the same test, could also be used to establish stability.

**c** Alternate forms would be better if the test taker is likely to remember and be influenced by the items or the answers from the first test.

## ACTIVITY FOUR

**a** Split-half reliability

**b** Cronbach's alpha

**c** Item-total correlation

**d** Kuder-Richardson (KR-20) coefficient

## ACTIVITY FIVE

Inter-rater reliability

## ACTIVITY SIX

**a** The reliability of 0.89 and 0.90 in this study exceeds the standard of 0.80 and would be considered adequate for this instrument.

**b** The first measurement was to assess anxiety in relation to the approaching surgery.

The second measurement was to assess anxiety in relation to affective pain after ambulation post-surgery. You would not expect a high correlation between the two measures because they are measuring anxiety in different contexts.

**c** No, the author acknowledged this limitation, but stated that 'the presence of verbal anchors was expected to enhance accuracy in surgical patients'. Therefore, the adequacy of the reliability for this measure is questionable.

# Chapter 13

## ACTIVITY ONE

**a** Data collection
- Written or oral data may be collected.
- Collect data through audiotaped and transcribed interviews and skilled observations.
- Participant observation, immersion, informant interviews.
- Use of primary and secondary data sources.

**b** Data analysis
- Move from participant's description to researcher synthesis.
- Data collection and analysis occur simultaneously, use theoretical sampling, constant-comparative method and axial coding.
- Data are collected and analysed simultaneously, searching for symbolic categories.
- Analyse for importance and then validity (authenticity) and reliability.

**c** Describing the findings
- A narrative elaboration of the lived experience.
- Descriptive language to show theory connection to the data.
- Large quantities of data, provide examples from the data and propositions about relationships of phenomena.
- Well-synthesised chronicle.

## ACTIVITY TWO

**a** Semi-structured interviews.
**b** Identification of themes.
**c** An integration of field notes and interviews.

## ACTIVITY THREE

**a** By ensuring that the criteria of credibility, auditability and fittingness have been met. Confirmability is then ensured.

**b** Barclay et al. (1996) stated that the 'Initial classification and the emerging analysis was "tested" by members of the research team who taught a weekly class of pregnant couples and by participants who confirmed the researchers' developing insights in further group discussions. The analysis was then verified by a group of eight men who were from another class and not involved in the focus groups'. Comparison of the findings with another study in another city 'provided valuable insights and … repeated examination of the literature' ensured theoretical sensitivity.

Kermode (1995) provided an outline of the analysis to five participants in the study to ensure that researcher understanding and interpretation of the data were compatible with the participants. Kermode also sought impressions of the analysis from four people with AIDS who were not involved in the study, and who confirmed the commonality of experiences.

### ACTIVITY FOUR

Triangulation is the process of combining two or more data sources, investigators, theories, and/or methods in a single study. It can also mean that studies can be conducted sequentially. For example, a qualitative study that describes a particular phenomenon can be followed by a quantitative study that adapts the themes and categories into variables/items in a questionnaire and is extended to a larger subject sample.

### ACTIVITY FIVE

Students will have different answers to this activity.



## Chapter 14

### ACTIVITY ONE

**a** Ratio
**b** Ratio
**c** Ordinal
**d** Nominal, ordinal or interval
**e** Nominal
**f** Ordinal
**g** Ratio
**h** Nominal
**i** Interval

### ACTIVITY TWO

**a** Mood state: ordinal or interval. It is not uncommon for data collected with a Likert Scale to be treated as interval. When critiquing this issue, you must consider the ability to measure the quantity and equivalence of difference between the categories of the Likert Scale.
**b** Perceived health status: ordinal.
**c** Calories: ratio.
**d** Mother's age (ratio); trimester of contact (nominal or ordinal); and birthweight (ratio).

### ACTIVITY THREE

**a** Mood state; only the first line of the table.
**b** Mean; standard deviation; study range; possible range (of instrument).
**c** Interval or ratio.
**d** Yes.

## ACTIVITY FOUR

**a** Yes. Means and standard deviations are used with interval or ratio data. Calories are measured at the ratio level.

**b** The mean number of calories consumed daily for the seventy-eight adolescent males was 3,322. The lowest number of daily calories consumed was 435; the greatest number of calories consumed was 7,753. If it is assumed that the distribution of calories consumed fits a normal distribution, then 68 per cent of the subjects consumed between 2,059 and 4,585 calories daily (mean $\pm$1 SD = 3,322 $\pm$ 1263 calories).

## ACTIVITY FIVE

**a** 41 subjects

**b** 31.71 years $\pm$ (2 SD $\times$ 7.29) = 31.71 $\pm$ 14.58; 95 per cent of the sample were aged between 17.13 and 46.29 years.

**c** 32 per cent

**d** The sample of forty-one participants were on average aged 31.7 years with twelve years of schooling and an annual family income of $9300. The sample had a mean of 1.3 children at home; were diagnosed over thirty months ago; and were on more than three prescribed medications. The majority of the sample were of African/American background, with a church affiliation, divorced or single, and were unemployed for the last thirteen months.

**e** The standard deviations for a number of variables are high; for example: time since last employment; annual family income; time since diagnosis; number of prescribed medications. This high variance would indicate that the distribution of scores are not of a normal (bell) shape (see page 376 of the textbook).

**f** A frequency distribution of all scores for each variable could be constructed and examined to see whether the mean is the most appropriate summary statistic; the mean and median scores of each variable could be compared. The median score is located towards the peak of the distribution, and its relationship to the mean indicates the skewness of the distribution (see page 377 of the textbook).

## ACTIVITY SIX

**a** 142.63

**b** Wives; Total problem score for CFIDS symptoms.

**c** The wives' score in Self Ability of Marital Empathy.

**d** Husbands

**e** Yes, the table and narrative agree.

## ACTIVITY SEVEN

Assuming a normal distribution, 68 per cent of patients in Clinic 1 would be seen between thirty to fifty minutes, while patients in Clinic 2 would be between zero and seventy minutes. The lower variation in Clinic 1 would be more tolerable for waiting. It would be useful to examine the frequency distribution for the waiting time of each clinic, particularly the frequencies for waiting times lower than the mean for Clinic 2 (that is less than twenty-five minutes).

## ACTIVITY EIGHT

- **a** mean  **b** range
- **c** median  **d** kurtosis
- **e** SD  **f** standard deviation
- **g** mode  **h** homogeneous
- **i** skewed

## ACTIVITY NINE

**a** Barclay et al. (1996): No
Waldenström and Nilsson (1994): Yes
Kermode (1995): No
Dracup et al. (1997): Yes

**b** Barclay et al. (1996): Yes
Waldenström and Nilsson (1994): Yes
Kermode (1995): Yes
Dracup et al. (1997): Yes

**c** Barclay et al. (1996): Demographic characteristics – age, duration of relationship, level of education, occupation.
Waldenström and Nilsson (1994): Demographic and clinical characteristics – age, length of gestation, parity, relationship, ethnic background, years of education; attitudes to breast feeding.
Kermode (1995): Demographic and clinical characteristics – age, length of hospital stay, AIDS-defining illness.
Dracup et al. (1997): Demographic and clinical characteristics – age, years of education, income, previous history, hospital delay time, thrombolytic therapy.

**d** Barclay et al. (1996): Yes, demographic description of the qualitative sample was appropriate.
Waldenström and Nilsson (1994): Yes
Kermode (1995): Yes, demographic and some clinical description of the qualitative sample was appropriate.
Dracup et al. (1997): Yes



# Chapter 15

## ACTIVITY ONE

This study has a critique provided in Chapter 18 of the textbook.

**a** See hypotheses and/or research questions (page 465 of the textbook).
**b** See hypotheses and/or research questions (page 465 of the textbook).
**c** See analysis section (page 468 of the textbook).
**d** See analysis section (page 468 of the textbook).

### ACTIVITY TWO

**a** Was there any difference in the duration and experience of breast feeding for women in birth centre care when compared to standard obstetric care?

**b** The research hypothesis was implied in the paper; a general statement, referred to as an hypothesis, was stated in the last paragraph of the introduction section, but there were no dependent variables listed.

**c** The level of measurement for these variables (parity, civil status and ethnic background) is nominal and presented as a percentage (%); the appropriate test is the chi-square ($\chi^2$), a non-parametric statistic.

**d** These variables were at the interval or ratio level, with two groups (levels of the independent variable) – see Table 15.1 on page 395 of the textbook.

**e** Eighty-three per cent of the experimental group participated in the antenatal education, while only 64 per cent participated from the control group; this was a statistically significant difference.

**f** t-test.

### ACTIVITY THREE

**a** There is an inverse relationship between the two variables.

**b** There are statistically significant inversely related correlations for self-efficacy and: 1) symptoms; and 2) duration of HIV-illness.

**c** This level of significance indicates a probability that the researcher would obtain a result by chance only 1 time in 1000. This is a highly significant finding.



### ACTIVITY FOUR

**a** What were the factors that affect patients' delay in seeking treatment following symptoms of acute myocardial infarction?

**b** Years of education; income; use of ambulance.

**c** Sex; age; ethnicity; location where symptoms occurred.

**d** Years of education; intermittent symptoms; not wanting to trouble anyone; symptoms seen as not serious; symptom of dizziness.

## Chapter 16

### ACTIVITY ONE

| | | |
|---|---|---|
| **a** False | **b** True | **c** False |
| **d** True | **e** True | **f** True |

### ACTIVITY TWO

The advice given should be based on whatever research evidence is available. From the Waldenström and Nilsson (1994) study however, it should be pointed out that women who gave birth at the birth centre seemed to need less obstetric medication in labour, they went home earlier, and they experienced greater support from the midwife during labour than those in standard care. In addition, they were more satisfied with the care they received during pregnancy, labour and after the birth. However, it also needs to be pointed out that women who gave birth in the birth centre experienced a greater incidence of sore nipples and milk stasis than those in standard care. The authors suggest several reasons for this finding which are plausible. For example, women in the birth centre may have been more inclined to report their experiences and symptoms, and it is possible that staff in the birth centre may have been less qualified to give breast-feeding support. Further research is needed in this area but it might be necessary to establish the experience of the midwives in regard to breast feeding before making a decision about where to give birth. Notwithstanding these findings, if women are highly motivated to breast feed, it doesn't matter where they give birth, and the site of pregnancy care, labour and post-partum has no effect on the duration of breast feeding.

## ACTIVITY THREE

**a** It means that women in the experimental group had a significantly shorter hospital stay than women in the control group.

**b** It can be concluded that there was no difference between the two groups in regard to the use of a breast pump at two months post-partum.

**c** Women in both groups were sent a questionnaire two months after delivery which included a question about the experience of the midwife in terms of the level of support given during labour. The question required respondents to indicate on a Likert-type Scale from 1 = no support at all, to 7 = extensive support. The result indicates that women in the experimental group received significantly more support from the midwife than women in the standard care group.



## ACTIVITY FOUR

**a** Measure of relationship between one interval level dependent variable and several independent variables

**b** Probability level

**c** Sample size

**d** Student's t-test

## ACTIVITY FIVE

True

## ACTIVITY SIX

**a** An audit trail is the researcher's development of the research process in a qualitative study that allows the reader (and other researchers) to follow the thinking or conclusions of the researcher. Barclay et al. (1996) use an audit trail to provide an insight into their thinking. They illustrate how the conceptual categories were established and how they related to the concepts identified in the data and the core category of 'confusion'.

**b** They used direct quotes from the participants to exemplify and support their interpretation of the data and the definition of categories.

**c** 'Confusion' is a finding that emerged as a core or central category because it is reflected in all the other categories that were identified except one.

**d** The conceptual model depicts diagrammatically the relationship between the categories identified from the data. It shows that 'anxiety' has elements of 'separation' and 'ambivalence', and that the category of 'need to know' intersects with 'ambivalence', 'adjustment' and 'development'. All of the categories, except 'development' are linked to the core category of 'confusion'. However, it is interesting to note that the audit trail figure does depict a relationship between 'development' and 'confusion'.

**e** From the findings of this study there are a number of implications for the practice of midwifery, most notably that first-time fathers need to know what to expect. The importance of developing interventions that are directed towards reducing the confusion experienced by these men is clearly evident. The finding that most men simply endured the antenatal classes, often resenting the ways in which information was provided, implies that the way in which the classes are conducted requires review. The sense of sharing the pregnancy experience with their partners is missing and greater emphasis on addressing the needs of this important group is necessary. As the authors point out, health professionals need to re-think their priorities if their goals are to prepare couples for parenthood and strengthen relationships into which babies are born.



**f** Several suggestions for further research are apparent from this work, including a comparative study of men who are confused by their partner's pregnancy and those who see it as a time for growth and development. A randomised controlled trial involving an experimental group who are exposed to antenatal classes that address the needs of men as well as women would be useful to establish a cause and effect relationship. An investigation that involves midwives' perceptions and attitudes could be undertaken to determine whether this variable could influence the men's experiences, and the women themselves could be studied for their views on how their partners are dealing with the event of pregnancy and the impact on relationships.

## ACTIVITY SEVEN

### *Box 1*

**a** Mean hours is the average number of hours for each variable from symptom onset to arrival at hospital. The median is the number of hours for each variable which divides the individual times into two equal groups. The table gives the upper and lower quartiles for each variable, that is the upper quartile being the point below which 75 per cent of the observed hours fall (for example, in the variable of Income and those who earned <$20,000, it is 26.6 hours), and the lower quartile is the point at which 25 per cent of the observed hours fall (in the variable of <$20,000 income, it is 2.5 hours).

Thus the interquartile range represents the middle 50 per cent of the study population, and means, for example, that 50 per cent of the subjects who earned less than $20,000 a year took between 2.5 and 26.6 hours to seek treatment for their cardiac symptoms. This measure is used in conjunction with the median to describe the centre and dispersion of ordinal data or interval/ratio level data that are skewed.

**b** Less than nine years.

**c** People who earned less than $20,000 per year delayed significantly longer in seeking treatment for MI symptoms than those who earned an annual income of greater than $60,000.

**d** The symbol for 'less than' (<) is inaccurate for the twelve years entry under Education, and the $60,000 entry under Income. Both should have the symbol for 'greater than' (>).

***Box 2***

**a** 'Too embarrassed to ask for assistance' (p= 0.007).

**b** 68 per cent

**c** Three social/cognitive factors were most significant (p=0.001) in relation to the time taken to respond to cardiac symptoms. The results show that significantly less people knew about the nature of cardiac symptoms; failed to realise the importance of their symptoms; and waited to see if the symptoms would go away. Each of these factors were significantly more likely to increase the delay time in seeking treatment than the other variables.



**d** Future nursing research could involve studies that explore the impact of educational programs and/or counselling strategies designed to improve knowledge and understanding of cardiac symptoms and the importance of seeking treatment early.

***Box 3***

**a** The variable 'symptoms seen as not serious', with an odds ratio of 1.40, is associated with a delay of greater than two hours in seeking treatment, whereas the variable 'symptom of dizziness', with an odds ratio of .33, is associated with a delay time of less than two hours.

**b** There is a significant relationship between people who experience intermittent cardiac symptoms and a delay time to seek treatment of greater than two hours.

**c** Years of education. From this study it can be predicted that people who have less than ten years of education are more likely to delay seeking treatment for cardiac symptoms. This factor is not amenable to nursing intervention.

**d** 0.05

## ACTIVITY EIGHT

Several implications for nursing practice can be identified from this study. They include a greater role in the provision of information to, and guidance for, individuals who experience a myocardial infarction. The authors identify that counselling strategies that prepare people for certain signs and symptoms will result in less delay in seeking treatment.

The provision of health education programs that promote an awareness of the nature of MI signs and symptoms and the rationale for seeking early treatment, by emphasising the effectiveness of thrombolytic therapies, would benefit members of the community.

## ACTIVITY NINE

**a** To explore the perceptions of patients with an AIDS-defining illness as they relate to nursing interventions that were helpful and unhelpful during their hospitalisation. A secondary aim, or purpose, was to develop an understanding of the human experience of being diagnosed with AIDS.

**b** The author states that themes were identified from the data using Colaizzi's method of analysis but does not provide any insights into the way in which this was done. It would have been more useful to briefly summarise the main aspects of this method for those who may be unfamiliar with Colaizzi's work.

**c** Three themes were identified in Table 1: The meaning of AIDS, nursing interventions, and the hospital experience. However, only data relating to the theme of nursing interventions, with the categories of care and carelessness, were presented in the text, as expected from the title and opening comments. Under the subheading of 'The Study' the author stated that only a brief summary of the experience of being diagnosed with AIDS ('The meaning of AIDS') would be reported in the article and this appears in the first paragraph under the heading 'Findings'. There is no reference to the theme of the hospital experience incorporating the categories of 'Intrusion' and 'Inadequacy'.



**d** Benner, and Benner and Wrubel have conducted research and written extensively about the practice of nursing – the main focus of this study. Their concepts, competencies/domains and ideas have been used by Kermode to help interpret the data and contextualise the findings related to the nursing interventions theme, and the categories of 'Care' and 'Carelessness'.

**e** The participant's views and comments are appropriate exemplars that reflect the observations and interpretations of 'Care' and 'Carelessness' made by the researcher. On several occasions, however, excerpts of the interviewer/participant's conversation have been reproduced and the inclusion of comments by the interviewer, such as 'Yeah', 'Right' and 'Mmhm' could be seen as superfluous and probably unnecessary.

**f** This article is explicitly concerned with presenting the findings of data gathered about the helpful and unhelpful aspects of nursing practice as it relates to the care of a person with an AIDS-defining illness – as outlined in the beginning. It includes a brief paragraph which summarises the findings concerned with the experience of being diagnosed with AIDS. However, the implications for practice that have been provided seem to relate mainly to the experience of being diagnosed with AIDS, and suggestions for associated interventions, most of which have not been presented in the Findings section, for example, 'Supporting Hopefulness' and 'Responding to Denial'. Other implications do include some aspects of the data presented, but overall the implications for practice do not seem to flow directly from the study findings.

# Chapter 17

## ACTIVITY ONE

Answers will vary.

## ACTIVITY TWO

**a** Examples of factors to consider when deciding whether the findings are applicable to another group of men is the degree of similarity between those in the original study and the new group of interest. If there is much similarity in subject demographic characteristics then the findings might be fitting to apply. For example, Barclay et al. (1996) found that a small number of men in their study were 'more developed' than others. An important factor to always consider when applying qualitative findings is that individuals are unique and that findings which are applicable to groups may not necessarily be characteristic of specific individuals.

**b** Context bound findings are findings from qualitative studies that describe specific processes or particular phenomena that should be viewed from a contextual perspective. This context may have cultural, historical or traditional values and mores tied to a time and place that are specific to the population studied.

**c** The context in which the Barclay et al. study took place is specific to first-time expectant fathers in a current relationship who were attending antenatal classes with their partner, and to that extent should be viewed from a contextual perspective. By narrowing the selection factors for the subject, although the findings would still not be generalisable, greater group homogeneity increases the contextual commonality. The study could be replicated because first-time expectant fathers attending antenatal classes with their partners are not uncommon and therefore potentially accessible.

**d** The findings of this study support those of others that found that men have negative experiences during their partner's pregnancy. This contributes to the existing body of knowledge and helps to establish an area of need to be addressed by health professionals. The concepts and ideas that emerged from the data facilitate an understanding of the basis upon which the categories were developed and therefore contribute to the overall knowledge base. The researchers identified a contrast between the core categories of 'confusion' and 'development' and suggest further research is required in this area, which also represents a contribution to the existing body of knowledge.

**e** The categories that were identified in this study could be used as the basis for question/item development in a questionnaire. For example, first-time expectant fathers could respond to questions that ask them to indicate on a Likert-type scale their level of anxiety, their perceptions of how they are adjusting to their partner's pregnancy, their attitude towards their partner, their level of knowledge, and so on. Such an instrument could be distributed to a large subject sample and the results used as further evidence of the impact of being a first-time expectant father.

## ACTIVITY THREE

**a** Study design
**b** Study method
**c** Data analysis
**d** Subject selection
**e** Findings described
**f** Data analysis
**g** Application of findings
**h** Study design
**i** Study method

## ACTIVITY FOUR

**a** Credibility: The truth of the findings in this study were established through several sources: members of the research team who were also involved in teaching antenatal classes; the participants themselves; eight men who had similar backgrounds to the subjects but were not involved in the study; and comparison between the emerging findings and those of another similar study.

**b** Auditability: A 'simplified' audit trail of the concept to core category analyses is provided, and enables the reader to follow the process of identifying concepts from the raw data, through the various steps of analysis to the interpretation of the findings.

**c** Fittingness: This study has remained true to the everyday reality of the participants. Their experiences are described in enough detail to allow other members of the profession to evaluate the findings and their applicability to other settings, as well as research and theory development. The authors also discussed their findings in the context of other research studies in the area.

## ACTIVITY FIVE

**a** Yes
**b** Yes
**c** No
**d** Yes
**e** Yes
**f** Yes
**g** Yes
**h** Yes
**i** Yes
**j** Yes



## ACTIVITY SIX

Several areas of concern might be identified and there are not necessarily singular answers that are right or wrong. Three examples are provided as a way to consider the value of the knowledge generated by the study; two concerns are related to the study participants and one is related to data collection.

First, the twenty years since the war may have affected the perceptions these nurses had about their experience and their responses may have been very different from what might have been expressed more immediately following their return from Vietnam.

Second, the fact that the majority of these nurses volunteered might make this population of nurses very different from a population that may not have had a choice. For instance, in more recent times nurses in the USA National Guard were called up and given orders to leave for Desert Storm within a week and had little time to prepare for the experience. It might have been a very different war experience than one where nurses who volunteered had the opportunity to consider the decision and make a choice. Different populations might identify different meanings of nursing wartime experiences.

A third concern is related to the questions asked during data collection. Other questions may have provided different knowledge and perhaps have been more important in understanding nursing during the war, including questions such as: (1) What were the difficult things you encountered while practising nursing in a wartime setting?, (2) Tell me about how the basic concepts of nursing differed? and (3) What ways do you think doing wartime nursing affected your nursing career and practice?

Because the majority of these nurses responded so long after the war experience, questions such as these might have built greater knowledge about ways nursing during a war experience affected later practice.

Critique of a qualitative study allows the persons evaluating the work to consider what might have been learned had the study been designed differently, and compare the current findings with the value of what might have been learned using alternative methods. Critique does not necessarily mean what was done or discovered was wrong, but allows the chance to view alternative methods for future research, think about what the investigator really wants to learn given the limitations of the study, think about the generalisability of the findings, and evaluate the knowledge learned.

# Chapter 18

## ACTIVITY ONE

A critique of the Good (1995) paper is provided on pages 464–9 of the textbook.



## ACTIVITY TWO

A critique of the Sharts-Hopko et al. (1996) paper is provided on pages 480–6 of the textbook.

# Chapter 19

## ACTIVITY ONE

**a** Yes

**b** Geritz (1992) examined 150 peripheral IV lock sites, Shoaf and Oliver (1992) examined 260 adult surgical patients, and Peterson and Kirchhoff (1991) included twenty studies in a meta-analysis. Of these twenty studies, nineteen focused on adult subjects. The patients are relatively comparable, although Geritz (1992) has a smaller sample size.

**c** All three studies are comparing similar flush protocols (independent variable), and the effect on patency and phlebitis (dependent variables).

**d** All three studies concluded there was no difference in patency or phlebitis when comparing flushing protocols.

**e** Yes, because no difference in outcomes were found between the two flush solutions and saline costs less. Normal saline.

**f** From the information available, Geritz (1992) seemed to be the only researcher who compared cost.

## ACTIVITY TWO

Answers will vary depending on the clinical setting.

## ACTIVITY THREE

**a** At many institutions a doctor orders the flush solution for IVs. Pharmacy may be involved in stocking, labelling, and preparing flush solutions. Therefore, it would be beneficial to include representatives from nursing, medicine and pharmacy. Different departments may request including their own representatives in any discussions of this practice change. Having department heads or other people in positions of authority appoint representatives rather than depending on volunteers will add value to the endeavour.

**b** Some representatives will accept your information at face value. However, to prevent any opposition from the beginning, it may be advisable to prepare the summary table, and distribute it as well as copies of the articles.

**c** In this example, cost effectiveness may be demonstrated by calculating supplies and staff time costs. However, an intervention may initially cost more in time and supplies, yet cost less overall due to improved clinical outcomes.

**d** It is important to proceed through the appropriate channels in your institution. Policies and procedures should be written to reflect the practice change. Communication to all departments affected is essential, possibly both in writing and presentation at departmental meetings. Sometimes the communication may be through the departmental representatives who were appointed earlier. Education for all staff affected should be thorough and include all shifts and units. Concise written information should be available on the practice change in areas that staff frequent. Individual unit representatives could be educated in depth and would then be available in the unit for questions and education.



**e** After implementation of the practice change it is important to assess compliance and watch for potential adverse events. For example, what are patency and phlebitis rates for the saline flush only when compared with rates prior to the change in flush solutions?

## ACTIVITY FOUR

**a** D; D; D; D

**b–g** Answers will vary depending on the clinical setting.